D1621272

The Big Prostate

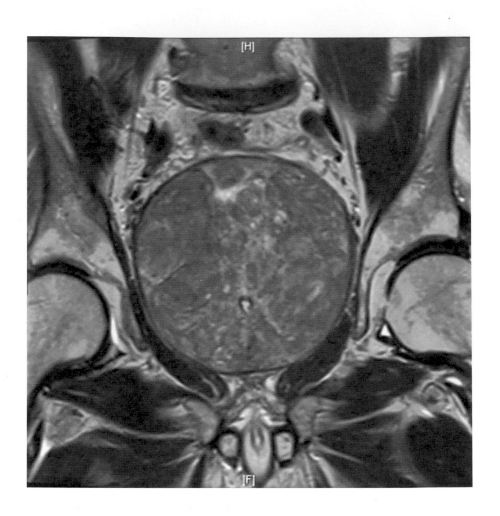

Veeru Kasivisvanathan • Ben Challacombe

Editors

The Big Prostate

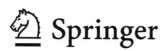

Editors
Veeru Kasivisvanathan
University College London & University
  College London Hospital
London, United Kingdom

Ben Challacombe
Guy's and St Thomas's Hospitals NHS
  Foundation Trust
London, United Kingdom

ISBN 978-3-319-64703-6   ISBN 978-3-319-64704-3   (eBook)
https://doi.org/10.1007/978-3-319-64704-3

Library of Congress Control Number: 2017958787

Printed on acid-free paper

This Springer imprint is published by Springer Nature
The registered company is Springer International Publishing AG
The registered company address is: Gewerbestrasse 11, 6330 Cham, Switzerland

Preface

With increasing life expectancy throughout populations globally, men have a greater chance of developing significant benign prostatic hyperplasia (BPH) than ever before. These men can present to urological services in a number of ways, some being referred by their primary care practitioners to secondary care with lower urinary tract symptoms, and others, presenting as an emergency directly to hospital services. Increasingly, those with larger prostates are being referred from secondary to tertiary care centres where specific technology may be available for the management of this problem.

There are a number of well-established medical, interventional and surgical management options available, but men with a particularly large prostate, over 100 cc, pose a particular challenge to clinicians. The big prostate is difficult to manage from the point of view of the complexity of presentation, pharmacological treatments, bleeding, catheterization, surgery and subsequent complications. This interesting group of men is one that all urologists involved in general urology will have encountered. However, there is a lack of guidance and resources dedicated specifically to the management of men with these huge prostates greater than 100 cc, which differs from the routine management of BPH in smaller glands.

This book will be of particular use to healthcare practitioners who manage men with BPH in the outpatient or emergency setting and in the operating theatre who want further tips on how to deal with the big prostate greater than 100 cc. It covers the anatomy and physiology of the big prostate, how it presents to medical services and the diagnostic challenges of raised prostate specific antigen testing in the big prostate. Medical treatment, which is commonly first line in benign prostatic hyperplasia, may not be as effective in the particularly large prostate and a chapter is dedicated to the evidence behind medical management in the big prostate.

The specific techniques, advantages and disadvantages of different surgical approaches specifically for the bigger prostates will be discussed. Prominent experts in the field will divulge intraoperative tips on surgical techniques from their years of experience for dealing with the huge gland. Prostate artery embolization, enucleation of the prostate, green light laser, transurethral resection of the prostate, simple robotic prostatectomy and open surgery are covered in dedicated chapters. There is a discussion on the management of the comorbid patient, which we are increasingly faced with, as well as advice on carrying out other non-BPH-related urological procedures in men who have a particularly difficult operation due to an obstructing big prostate. The book will be rounded off by a discussion on what the future holds for the management of huge BPH.

In summary, huge BPH is a growing problem which may become an increasingly common presentation in future years. We believe that all urologists, trainees, emergency medicine doctors, primary care doctors and medical students interested in men's health will greatly benefit from the information, advice and techniques covered in this first book dedicated to the Big Prostate.

London, UK   Veeru Kasivisvanathan
London, UK   Ben Challacombe

Contents

Chapter 1
Anatomy, Physiology and Pathology of the Large Prostate

Osayuki Nehikhare, Veeru Kasivisvanathan, Harold Ellis, and Ben Challacombe

1.1 Anatomy of the Large Prostate

The male prostate is a derivative of the primitive endoderm, developing during embryogenesis from the cloaca. The connected vas deferens and seminal vesicles develop from the mesonephric ducts, which secrete fluid which comprise semen. The prostate is a fibromuscular gland, pyramidal in shape and surrounding the male urethra. It is surrounded by peri-prostatic fascia. A thin layer of connective tissue forms the true capsule. Superficial to the true capsule is the pseudocapsule, formed by three layers of fascia on the anterior, posterior and lateral aspect of the prostate. Superiorly, the gland is continuous with the bladder neck. The urethra enters the base of the prostate from the anterior border. Inferiorly, the apex of the gland lies on the external sphincter of the bladder (Fig. 1.1).

O. Nehikhare (✉)
University Hospital Coventry & Warwickshire NHS Trust, Coventry, UK

University College London Hospital, London, UK

King's College London, London, UK

Guy's Hospital, London, UK
e-mail: osayuki.nehikhare@doctors.org.uk

V. Kasivisvanathan
University College London Hospital, London, UK
e-mail: veeru.kasi@ucl.ac.uk

H. Ellis
King's College London, London, UK

Guy's Hospital, London, UK
e-mail: harold.ellis@kcl.ac.uk

B. Challacombe
MRC Centre for Transplantation, King's College London, London, UK

Guy's Hospital, London, UK
e-mail: benchallacombe@doctors.org.uk

© Springer International Publishing AG 2018
V. Kasivisvanathan, B. Challacombe (eds.), *The Big Prostate*,
https://doi.org/10.1007/978-3-319-64704-3_1

1

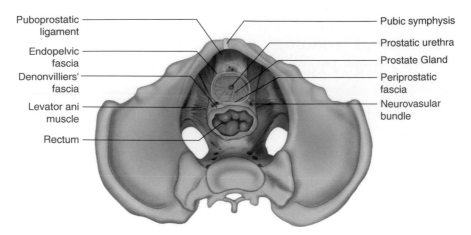

Fig. 1.1 Anatomy of the adult male pelvis illustrating the relationship prostate to the pelvic bones, neurovascular bundle and pelvic floor structures

Anterior to the prostate is the pubic symphysis, separated from it by the extra-peritoneal fat of the retro-pubic space (Cave of Retzius). Within this space lies the peri-prostatic plexus of veins. The puboprostatic ligaments connect the apex of the prostate to the pubis. The fascia of Denovilliers lies posterior to the prostate separating it from the rectum, whilst laterally is the levator ani muscle which fuses with the lateral fasia of the prostate [1].

The vas deferens and the seminal vesicles join to form the ejaculatory ducts at the supero-posterior part of the gland and open into the prostatic urethra on either side of the verumontanum.

1.1.1 Vascular Supply

The arterial blood supply is generally from the inferior vesical artery, a branch of the internal iliac artery, which enters the prostate from either side of the gland. Additional arterial supply can come from the middle rectal and pudendal arteries. The venous system forms a prostatic plexus, which receives the dorsal vein of the penis and drains into the internal iliac vein on each side of the gland (Fig. 1.2).

1.1.2 Neurological Innervation

The nerve supply of the prostate is from both the autonomic and somatic nervous systems. The autonomic, para-sympathetic (PS) innervation arises from sacral levels S2-S4. The PS nerves end at the acini cells of the prostate and lead to prostatic secretions. The sympathetic nerves supply originates from the thoraco-lumbar levels T12-L2 and produce contraction of the smooth muscle of the prosatic capsule

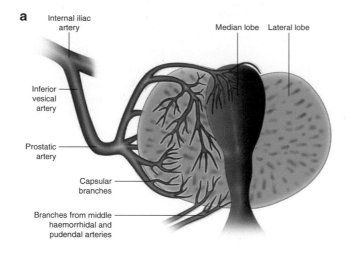

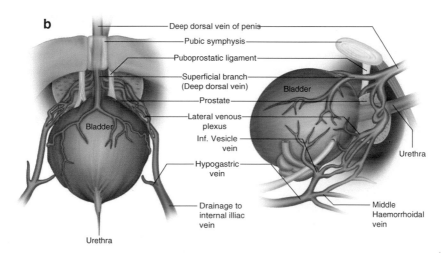

Fig. 1.2 (**a**) Arterial supply to the prostate derived from the internal iliac, inferior vesicle, middle rectal and pudendal arteries. (**b**) Prostate venous drainage. (*I*) Deep dorsal vein of the penis viewed from the rertopubic space. Relationship of the superficial venous branch and lateral plexus of veins is seen. (*II*) Lateral view of the pelvic venous plexus

and stroma. The main somatic innervation is from the pudendal nerve which innervates the striated sphincter and levator ani controlling the internal sphicter.

1.1.3   *Lymphatic Drainage*

The lymphatic drainage of the prostate is to the obturator and the internal iliac lymphatic nodes. There is also lymphatic communication to the external iliac, presacral, and the para-aortic lymph nodes.

1.1.4 Zones of the Prostate

In adults up to the age 50 the average prostate gland is approximately the size of a chestnut, 15–30 cc, enlarging by hypertrophy. However, a growing cohort of male patients are presenting with lower urinary tract symptoms (LUTS) in the context of a clinically large prostate greater than 100 cc. This provides a new clinical challenge in the management of their symptoms.

The prostate gland can be divided further into three zones: Transition zone (TZ), Central zone (CZ), and Peripheral zone (PZ) [2, 3]. The prostate consists of 70% glandular tissue and 30% fibromuscular stroma. The TZ accounts for 10% of the glandular tissue and 20% of adenocarcinomas (Fig. 1.3).

The TZ is where benign prostatic hyperplasia (BPH) occurs and can lead to bladder outflow obstruction (BOO) if the adenoma grows large enough to narrow or compress the prostatic urethra. The TZ is often described as having two lateral lobes and a median lobe that can lead to the symptoms of the lower urinary tract symptoms (LUTS).

A urethral crest runs along the posterior midline and disappears at the membranous urethra. On both sides of the urethral crest, there is a grove where the prostatic sinuses exist and drain all of the glandular elements. The urethral crest widens and protrudes from the posterior wall as the seminal colliculus (verumontanum). A small midline pit, the prostatic utricle, is found at the apex of the seminal colliculus. On either side of the utricular orifice, the small slit like openings to the ejaculatory duct can be found.

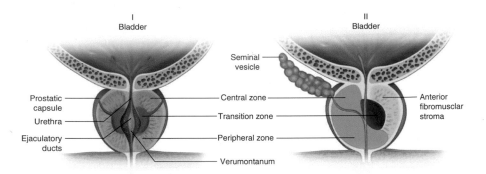

Fig. 1.3 Anatomical zones of the prostate and their relationship to the bladder, seminal vesicles and urethra. (*I*) Cross sectional view illustrating, TZ—bilateral regions in the middle to the base of the gland, (along the proximal urethra), composed of ducts extending laterally from the urethral wall and curving anteromedially; (*II*) Sagittal view of prostate illustrating CZ —a flattened conical structure with ducts branching from the verumontanum (mid-prostate) to the prostatic base and surrounding the seminal vesicles; Anterior fibromuscular stroma, a wedge-shaped stromal barrier, occupying much of the anteromedial prostatic tissue. PZ—The major glandular component of the prostate, extending from the urethra at the verumontanum to the prostatic apex

The CZ is the area surrounding the ejaculatory ducts. This zone consists of 25% of the glandular tissue. Very few adenocarcinomas are found in this region and can represent as little as 1–5% of tumours in the prostate.

The PZ of the prostate constitutes 70% of the glandular tissue. This zone covers the posterior and lateral aspects of the prostate. The peripheral zone is the area that is palpated on digital rectal examination (DRE) and represents the area where 70% of adenocarcinomas are found. This area is also the location most commonly affected by chronic prostatitis [4].

1.2   Physiology of the Large Prostate

The principal function of the prostate is to provide the proteins and electrolytes that form the bulk of the seminal fluid. Furthermore, the prostate has a role in maintaining continence through autonomic control of the internal urethral sphincter. In men with BPH, the enlarged prostate presses against the urethra. The bladder wall becomes thickened form hyperplasia of the muscle fibres of the bladder wall and eventually the bladder may weaken and lose the ability to empty, leaving some urine in the bladder. The combination of narrowing of the urethra and incomplete emptying of the bladder can lead to urinary incontinence through secondary detrusor overactivity.

The adult human prostate is a tubuloalveolar gland composed of ducts lined with pseudo-stratified columnar epithelium. The cells lining the ducts are columnar and secretory, with basal nuclei. An almost continuous layer of basal epithelial cells forms the basement membrane. The prostatic epithelium is, in turn, surrounded by a dense fibromuscular stroma.

The embrylogical development of the prostate begins with the growth of prostatic buds from the urogenital sinus at about 10 weeks of fetal development in humans. Androgen receptors (AR) in the urogenital sinus are stimulated by testicular androgens to induce epithelial budding, proliferation and differentiation, to form the ductal structures.

In the mature prostate androgens are believed to act upon the prostatic smooth muscle (which expresses AR) to maintain a fully differentiated, growth-quiescent epithelium. This occurs via stromal–epithelial cell interactions under the control of regulatory growth factors.

BPH is characterised by an increase in both epithelial and stromal cell numbers of the prostate. During embryological development there is formation of new prostatic glands. However, the development of new glands in the adult prostate has given rise to the hypothesis of "re-awakening" of proliferating cells. This increase in cell number could be due to proliferation of stromal and epithelial cells, as well as impairment of programmed cell death [5].

1.2.1 Testosterone

It has long been recognised that testosterone leads to prostate growth and with increasing age in men, BPH, which is linked, to BOO and LUTS. Cell proliferation within the prostate is controlled by testosterone. Testosterone can bind directly to the androgen receptor (AR), or may be converted to its more potent form, dihydrotestoterone (DHT) by the hormone 5α-reductase (5AR) [6].

Testosterone diffuses into both epithelial and prostatic stromal cells. In epithelial cells it binds directly to the AR. In prostate stromal cells the majority of testosterone binds directly to the 5AR hormone and is converted to DHT, which then binds with more affinity and thus more potency to the AR than in the stromal cells.

The hormone-receptor complex then interacts with cell DNA at specific binding sites inducing transcription of 5AR mRNA and subsequent protein synthesis [7].

There are two isoforms of 5AR: Type-I 5AR, which is found in the liver, skin and prostate and Type-II 5AR, found predominantly in the prostate stromal cells but not within the prostatic epithelial cells.

This has clinical and pharmacological significance as Finasteride is selective for type-I 5AR whereas Dutasteride inhibits both type-I and type-II 5AR [8].

Studies demonstrate that 5AR Type-I and Type-II mRNA are present in all prostate zones, including the PZ, TZ and CZ, in tissue samples from individuals with a normal prostate, patients with BPH and patients with prostate cancer.

Patients with large prostates have an increased risk of concomitant BPH and prostate cancer (PCa). Large glands with BPH have been shown to have an increased expression of 5-AR Types I and II mRNA. In PCa, Type-I 5AR mRNA is overexpressed but Type-II is not [9].

1.2.2 Androgen Hypothesis

Historically it was believed that PCa was related to testosterone levels. Thus the 'Androgen Hypothesis" was used to explain relationship that high levels of testosterone predispose patients to PCa and low levels of testosterone were protective. However, the androgen hypothesis has been seriously challenged, as overwhelming evidence contradicts its basic principles [6]. Evidence shows that men with high serum testosterone are not at an increased risk of developing PCa and that low serum testosterone provides no protection against the development of PCa. Furthermore some men with untreated PCa can receive testosterone therapy without subsequent risk of PCa progression [7].

The androgen hypothesis has therefore been replaced by the 'Saturation Model', whereby the prostate tissue is shown to be sensitive to changes of testosterone at low levels but indifferent above a set threshold. This threshold effect occurs when increasing androgen levels reach a limit beyond which there is no further ability to induce androgen driven changes to prostate tissue [10].

1.2.3   Growth Factors

As well as androgens, other soluble modulators have an effect on the prostate tissue. Stromal and epithelial cell interactions are mediated by soluble growth factors, which stimulate or inhibit cell division and differentiation.

Growth stimulating factors include basic fibroblastic growth factor, epidermal growth factor, keratinocyte growth factor (KGF), and insulin-like growth factor (IGF). Transforming growth factors (TGFB) normally inhibit epithelial cell proliferation and it is possible that TGFB is down-regulated in BPH [11].

1.3   Pathology of the Large Prostate

BPH begins in the sub-mucosal layer of the TZ around the proximal urethra. There is proliferation of epithelial cells of the acini, ductules, smooth muscle and stromal fibroblasts. These changes, especially in larger prostates, cause distortion and compression of the urethra which results in LUTS (Table 1.1). Other complications of BPH occur less frequently than LUTs but may include acute urinary retention (AUR), renal failure, recurrent urinary tract infections (UTI's), haematuria and bladder stones.

The central prostate is also affected by benign prostatic enlargement, causing compression of the PZ and fibrosis, resulting in a surgical capsule. Increased urethral resistance results in compensatory changes in bladder function. Higher detrusor pressures are required to maintain urinary flow. Evidence suggests that men with larger prostates are at much higher risk of LUTS and their complications and benefit from early intervention from treatment to reduce the risk of long term complications [12].

Squamous metaplasia of the ductal epithelium at the PZ is common, especially in larger prostates, with 10–20% of patients having incidental foci of adenocarcinoma. 70% of prostate cancers develop in the PZ. The non-invasive proliferation of

Table 1.1 Summary of lower urinary tract symptoms (LUTS) grouped into storage and voiding LUTS

Storage LUTS	Voiding LUTS
Frequency	Hesitancy
Urgency	Poor stream
Nocturia	Intermittent dribbling
Incontinence	Terminal dribbling
Bladder pain	Strain on passing urine

epithelial cells within the ducts is termed prostatic intra-epithelial neoplasia (PIN). High grade PIN is generally considered to be a precursor of cancer though its clinical significance is more widely debated. 95% of prostate cancers are adenocarcinomas, with the remainder being ductal, squamous, transitional cell tumours and rarely carcinosarcomas [13].

1.3.1 Histology

Most prostatic adenocarcinomas are acinar in origin and feature small to medium-sized glands that lack organization and infiltrate the stroma. Progressive loss of differentiation of the prostatic adenocarcinoma is characterized by increasing variability in gland size and cell organization, as well as occurrence of papillary and cribiform patterns.

1.3.2 Cytology

On microscopic examination, prostate cancer cells show pleomorphic and hyperchromatic nuclei. Their cytoplasm is stained to become eosinophillic and there are have highly visible nuclei on a background of chromatin near the nuclear membrane.

1.3.3 Grading

Core biopsies are routinely taken for patients with abnormal DRE or raised prostate specific antigen (PSA). The histological aggressiveness of the disease is quantified using the modified Gleason grading system, in which the dominant and secondary histological patterns are scored from 3 (well differentiated) to 5 (undifferentiated), and summed up to a total score of 6–10 for each tumour [14, 15].

The best-differentiated tumours have a Gleason score of 6 (3 + 3), with well circumscribed glands but variation in shape and size, whereas undifferentiated cancers have a score of 10 (5 + 5) and show no glandular differentiation and central necrosis. When combined with the tumour stage, the Gleason grading system has a prognostic value, with lower scores correlating with a better prognosis [16]. There has been a recent proposal to change this into Gleason Grade Groups 1–5 which authors suggest are a simplified more accurate way of assigning risk of disease (Table 1.2). This new grading system was accepted by the World Health Organization (WHO) for the 2016 edition of Pathology and Genetics: Tumours of the Urinary System and Male Genital Organs [14].

Table 1.2 Gleason patterns of the modern Gleason grading system and the corresponding new grade group system

Gleason pattern	Gleason score	Grade group
3 Distinct, discrete individual glands	3 + 3 = 6	I
	3 + 4 = 7	II
4 Fused, cribriform or poorly formed glands	4 + 3 = 7	III
	4 + 4 = 8 3 + 5 = 8 5 + 3 = 8	IV
5 Necrosis, cords, sheets, solid nests	4 + 5 = 9 5 + 4 = 9 5 + 5 = 10	V

1.3.4   Invasion and Metastasis

The high frequency of invasion of the prostatic capsule by adenocarcinoma relates to the subcapsular location of tumours in the PZ. Perineural tumour invasion is common but presents a poor prognostic indicator. Peripheral nerves are devoid of lymphatics so contiguous spread of the tumour along tissue planes is the process of disease progression. Seminal vesicles can be involved, with bladder invasion occurring in advanced disease.

Prostate metastasis occurs early on in the disease, with dissemination to the iliac and para-aortic lymph nodes. Lymph node dissection (LND) during Robot Assisted Radical Prostatectomy (RARP) allows for accurate staging of PCa. The internal iliac, obturator, and lateral hypogastric lymph nodes commonly resected in high risk patients may decrease disease progression and potentially increase survival [17].

Lung metastasis reflects further lymphatic spread through the thoracic duct and dissemination from the prostatic venous plexus to the inferior vena-cava. As a consequence of haematological and lymphatic spread, bone metastases often occur, particularly to the skull vault, vertebral column, ribs, pelvic bones and the upper ends of the humerus and femur. These sites correspond to the distribution of the highly vascular red bone marrow.

1.4   Conclusion

With an increasing population of men possessing larger prostate glands there is a growing risk of more men suffering from LUTS and their complications. It is becoming more important for the clinical urologist to understand the affect of the large prostate and the relationship between the anatomy of the gland and the pathophysiology of both benign and malignant disease to improve the clinical management of patients.

References

1. Kim JH, Kinugasa Y, Hwang SE, Murakami G, Rodriguez-Vazquez JF, Cho BH. Denonvilliers' fascia revisited. Surg Radiol Anat. 2015;37(2):187–97.
2. McNeal JE. Origin and evolution of benign prostatic enlargement. Invest Urol. 1978;15(4):340–5.
3. McNeal JE, Kindrachuk RA, Freiha FS, Bostwick DG, Redwine EA, Stamey TA. Patterns of progression in prostate-cancer. Lancet. 1986;1(8472):60–3.
4. Fine SW, Reuter VE. Anatomy of the prostate revisited: implications for prostate biopsy and zonal origins of prostate cancer. Histopathology. 2012;60(1):142–52.
5. Isaacs JT, Coffey DS. Etiology and disease process of benign prostatic hyperplasia. Prostate. 1989:33–50.
6. Feldman HA, Longcope C, Derby CA, Johannes CB, Araujo AB, Coviello AD, et al. Age trends in the level of serum testosterone and other hormones in middle-aged men: Longitudinal results from the Massachusetts Male Aging Study. J Clin Endocrinol Metab. 2002;87(2):589–98.
7. Khera M, Crawford D, Morales A, Salonia A, Morgentaler A. A new era of testosterone and prostate cancer: from physiology to clinical implications. Eur Urol. 2014;65(1):115–23.
8. Andriole G, Bruchovsky N, Chung LWK, Matsumoto AM, Rittmaster R, Roehrborn C, et al. Dihydrotestosterone and the prostate: the scientific rationale for 5 alpha-reductase inhibitors in the treatment of benign prostatic hyperplasia. J Urol. 2004;172(4):1399–403.
9. Ho CKM, Habib FK. Estrogen and androgen signaling in the pathogenesis of BPH. Nat Rev Urol. 2011;8(1):29–41.
10. Morgentaler A, Traish AM. Shifting the paradigm of testosterone and prostate cancer: the saturation model and the limits of androgen-dependent growth. Eur Urol. 2009;55(2):310–21.
11. Chan JM, Stampfer MJ, Giovannucci E, Gann PH, Ma J, Wilkinson P, et al. Plasma insulin-like growth factor I and prostate cancer risk: A prospective study. Science. 1998;279(5350):563–6.
12. Emberton M, Fitzpatrick JM, Rees J. Risk stratification for benign prostatic hyperplasia (BPH) treatment. BJU Int. 2011;107(6):876–80.
13. Bostwick DG, Brawer MK. Prostatic intraepithelial neoplasia and early invasion in prostate-cancer. Cancer. 1987;59(4):788–94.
14. Epstein JI, Egevad L, Amin MB, Delahunt B, Srigley JR, Humphrey PA, et al. The 2014 International Society of Urological Pathology (ISUP) consensus conference on gleason grading of prostatic carcinoma definition of grading patterns and proposal for a new grading system. Am J Surg Pathol. 2016;40(2):244–52.
15. Epstein JI, Allsbrook WC, Amin MB, Egevad LL, Bastacky S, Beltran AL, et al. The 2005 International Society of Urological Pathology (ISUP) consensus conference on Gleason grading of prostatic carcinoma. Am J Surg Pathol. 2005;29(9):1228–42.
16. Kryvenko ON, Epstein JI. Prostate cancer grading a decade after the 2005 Modified Gleason Grading System. Arch Pathol Lab Med. 2016;140(10):1140–52.
17. van der Poel HG, Buckle T, Brouwer OR, Olmos RAV, van Leeuwen FWB. Intraoperative laparoscopic fluorescence guidance to the sentinel lymph node in prostate cancer patients: clinical proof of concept of an integrated functional imaging approach using a multimodal tracer. Eur Urol. 2011;60(4):826–33.

Chapter 2
Emergency and Elective Presentation of the Big Prostate

Oussama Elhage and Ben Challacombe

2.1 Introduction

The development of the very large prostate (>100 cc) is increasingly a recent phenomenon. In the previous decades prior to the introduction of medical therapy (mostly alpha blockers) for the symptoms of benign enlargement of the prostate and bladder outflow obstruction, the standard treatment was transurethral resection of the prostate. Therefore, most patients with an enlarged prostate who had symptoms were treated with an operation before their prostate reached large volumes. In the contemporary clinical practice, almost all patients are offered alpha blockers when they develop voiding symptoms. In the UK general practitioners can start treatment months or even years before the patient is referred to urologist [1].

Although androgens play an essential role in prostate development and growth in early adulthood [2, 3], there is however conflicting evidence of the effect of androgens on benign prostatic hyperplasia (BPH). It is suggested that the change in the testosterone/oestrogen ratio may play a role in the development of BPH [4]. The incidence of very large BPH remains very rare and most studies reporting the large prostate are case reports [5, 6]. The largest reported enlarged prostate is of the size of almost 4000cc [7]. This was measured on MRI and the report suggested it was treated conservatively. There is no consensus to what constitutes a very large prostate, some authors arbitrarily defined giant prostate hyperplasia for any gland measured above 200 g [8]. Most authors

O. Elhage (✉)
MRC Centre for Transplantation, King's College London, London, UK

The Urology Centre, Guy's & St Thomas NHS Foundation Trust, London, UK
e-mail: oussama.elhage@kcl.ac.uk

B. Challacombe
The Urology Centre, Guy's & St Thomas NHS Foundation Trust, London, UK
e-mail: benchallacombe@doctors.org.uk

© Springer International Publishing AG 2018
V. Kasivisvanathan, B. Challacombe (eds.), *The Big Prostate*,
https://doi.org/10.1007/978-3-319-64704-3_2

reporting the outcome on Holmium Enucleation of the Prostate (HoLEP) or simple prostatectomy as a surgical treatment for very large BPH use 80 cc as a cut off size [9, 10].

Obesity has been shown to be associated with BPH. In a study of more than 1600 patients, Bhindi et al found a direct correlation between increased body mass index and prostate size. For every 5 kg/m^2 increase in BMI, the authors found a 2.1 mL increase in prostate size [11]. In a mouse model, obesity was found to cause voiding dysfunction [12]. Metabolic syndrome is implicated in lower urinary tract symptoms and prostate enlargement [13, 14].

Very large BPH may cause variety of symptoms or none at all. Patients are usually not aware of how large their prostate is and can present to the urology clinic with symptoms of bladder outflow obstruction, however there are peculiarities specific to the very large prostate.

We will explore the different types of presentation in this chapter.

2.2   Emergency Presentations

Patients who have very large BPH often may not realise how large their gland is and are completely unaware of the implications of this. They may develop the typical symptoms of bladder outflow obstruction with voiding symptoms and are usually started on alpha blockers for some time before their presentation. Occasionally patients can present acutely with one of the following.

2.2.1   Haematuria

The enlarged prostate is usually extremely vascular. Around 2.5% of men with BPH will present with haematuria [15]. The incidence is expected to be higher in very large BPH. the patient may develop microscopic or macroscopic haematuria. The patient is usually alarmed after one episode of visible blood; however non-visible haematuria may require multiple visits to the general practitioner before it is investigated. This would eventually lead to referral to urological service where the typical investigation would conclude that the patient has bladder outflow obstruction and an enlarged prostate. Occasionally patients develop recurrent haematuria requiring multiple admissions. However, a careful assessment would reveal the cause of the bladder outflow obstruction to be an enlarged prostate. Without the aid of adequate imaging or due to the patients body habitus, the assessing urologist may underestimate the size of the prostate at physical examination [16] and there is hence a risk of only realising how large the prostate is on endoscopy just before the start of transurethral resection. Recurrent haematuria can be treated with a 5 alpha-reductase inhibitor such as finasteride or dutasteride but if a significant problem then a procedure may be required. The options in the setting of huge BPH are prostate artery embolisation (see Chap. 6) or if surgery is required then HoLEP, Greenlight PVP, TURP and open simple prostatectomy are also options.

2.2.2 Clot Retention

Patients with very large BPH often develop more significant and dangerous haematuria compared to other patients with smaller prostates. Not all patients who present with haematuria will require admission or a catheter insertion. Admission is recommended if a visible haematuria is associated with difficulty in voiding and if there is drop in Hb level, and in most patients with anticoagulants other than aspirin (warfarin, clopidogrel, heparin). Patients will require a three-way catheter insertion if the haematuria is severe with clots, and the patient is experiencing difficulty in voiding. three-way catheter is a specific type catheter with three channels; one for inflating the balloon, one channel for the inflow of the irrigating fluid and once channel for the outflow. Insertion of this catheter is no different to the insertion of all other catheters; however, it is recommended that a larger gauge catheter is inserted, at least size 20 ch. The typical practice is to insert 22ch three-way catheter in a patient with haematuria who requires irrigation. The irrigation system consists of bag of irrigation fluid (Saline), tubing system to connect it to the inflow opening of the three-way catheter. The outflow opening of the catheter is attached to a catheter draining bag. The fluid is infused slowly in the bladder and drained continually in the draining bag. The aim is to avoid accumulation of clots in the bladder which can cause further bleeding and severe patient distress and discomfort. Patients who develop clot retention at presentation will require three-way catheter insertion and a manual bladder washout should be performed. Some patients will require evacuation of clots under rigid cystoscopy and an anaesthetic. This can be a challenging procedure fraught with difficulty as the size of the prostate may limit the access to the bladder. An extra long resectoscope may be required and a series of Ellick evacuators and bladder syringes will be required to remove the bladder clots. Following this emergency procedure it is wise to consent the patient for urgent elective treatment such as HoLEP, open simple prostatectomy or PAE (see subsequent Chaps. 6–11) to prevent a recurrence.

2.2.3 Difficult Catheterisation

Not infrequently patients may require catheterisation for urine output or tissue perfusion monitoring purposes or perioperatively following non-urological major operations and patients who have large BPH may present a challenge for catheterisation to the non-expert. Often urologists are called to help with catheterising a patient

Fig. 2.1 In the large prostate, a common problem with catheterisation is to negotiate the acute angle and the high bladder neck. Standard catheters can fail to pass and may cause the formation of false passage. This may result in extreme difficulty in subsequent attempts at inserting a catheter

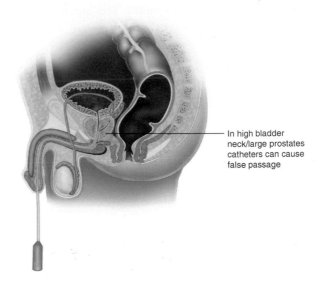

In high bladder neck/large prostates catheters can cause false passage

who otherwise didn't previously have symptoms only to find insertion of the catheter is difficult beyond the prostatic fossa due to the enlarged prostate (Fig. 2.1). In these cases, a curved tip catheter (16Fr, Tiemann or coudé tip) in case of bleeding can help negotiate the high bladder neck and middle lobe (Fig. 2.2). It is unwise to use a rigid introducer in these situations as a stricture or the prostate will lead to the formation of a false passage. One option is to pass a flexible guidewire down the urethra in the hope that it will gradually "find its way" into the bladder and then subsequently pass an open ended catheter over it. The safest and more secure way to catheterise in this situation is to use a flexible cystoscopy and directly pass a floppy guidewire under direct vision. Once the cystoscope is removed an open ended catheter is passed into the bladder.

2.2.4   Acute Urinary Retention

In a similar scenario to bladder outflow obstruction in enlarged prostate the very large prostate can cause bladder outflow obstruction and acute painful urinary retention. The patient would develop lower abdominal pain and inability to pass urine. the symptoms are usually identical to BPH except and in some cases, catheter insertion may prove to be difficult. Insertion of suprapubic catheter in these cases is fraught with danger as the part of the prostate may lie in the path of the suprapubic trocar and an unwitting insertion of such catheter my result in piercing of the prostate and subsequent catastrophic bleeding (Fig. 2.3). A radiologically guided insertion of suprapubic catheter in these cases is warranted. The likelihood of passing a

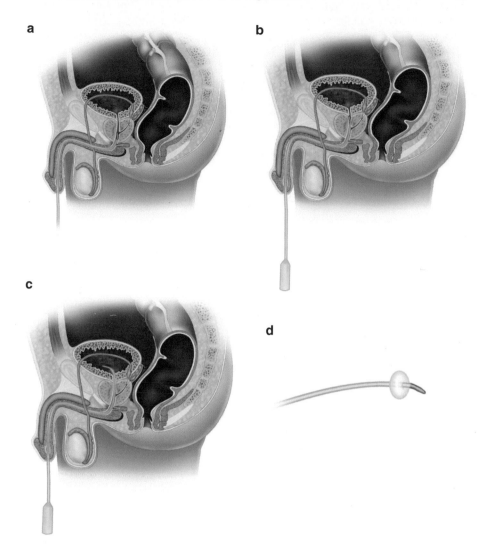

Fig. 2.2 (**a–d**) Tiemann tip catheter insertion in a patient with a large prostate. (**a–c**) The specially curved tip catheter is successfully able to negotiate the acute angle at the bladder neck and is passed into the bladder easily. (**d**) The shape of the tip of the catheter. Care should be taken when inserting this type of catheter as the concavity of the curve should face anteriorly otherwise a great deal of damage and false passage can be inflicted. Only a person who is familiar with this type of catheters and with the prostate anatomy should attempt at using it

trial of voiding is much less with a huge gland and therefore there should be a low threshold for moving onto bladder outflow surgery in these men. In addition to immediate failure to void following catheter removal, a subsequent episode of acute retention may lead to a difficult catheterisation and haematuria or the need to place-ment of a supra-pubic catheter thus pushing the urologist to operate sooner rather than later on these cases.

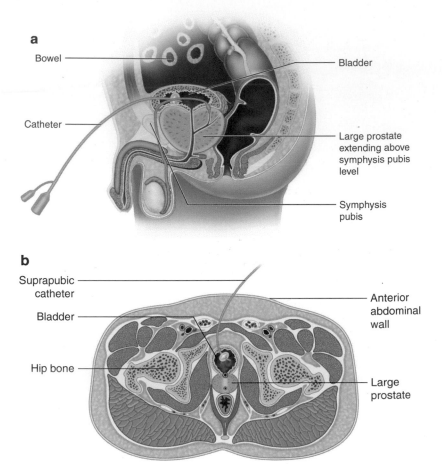

Fig. 2.3 (**a, b**) Insertion of suprapubic catheter in patient with large prostate can pause a huge challenge. (**a**) The prostate can be large enough and become an intra-abdominal organ. (**b**) A standard suprapubic catheter in this case is dangerous as it runs the risk of spearing the prostate which may result in catastrophic bleeding. To avoid the prostate, the surgeon may have to place the suprapubic catheter more proximally on the abdominal wall; this in turn run the risk of bowel injury. A more cautious approach would be to insert the suprapubic catheter in the interventional radiology suite under imaging guidance

2.2.5 Acute Renal Insufficiency

Occasionally some patients may present with signs of renal failure with high pressure urinary retention. These patients need urgent catheter insertion and acute management of their renal failure. Concurrent renal impairment can result from decreased GRF and can lead to abnormal creatinine. A scan of the urinary tract will usually reveal hydronephrosis. An urgent admission to the urology ward is required. This serves two purposes, first is to monitor and correct any diuresis which might ensue following catheterisation. Post catheterisation diuresis develop almost immediately following catheter insertion. A high urine output without adequate compensation in fluid intake would rapidly lead to dehydration and hypovolaemia, a dangerous state if the patient is at home. Therefore, all patient with suspected diuresis are kept in the hospital. Their vital signs and urine output should be monitored hourly in the first few hours of diuresis. However fluid replacement strategy should be based on average output over several hours rather than very short period. The typical replacement is normal oral fluid if the urine output is less than 200 ml/hr. The patient is usually able to drink one cup of fluid an hour. If the urine output is higher than 200 mL/h, an iv fluid replacement might be necessary with saline. Daily patient weight should be measured and recorded in a special log, this will give an indication if the fluid replacement is adequate. Blood electrolyte should be monitored daily till diuresis resolves.

The second purpose of admission is to monitor renal function. Blood creatinine level can initially rise sharply. The renal function typically improves to almost pre-retention level especially if the acute episode was treated promptly with catheterisation. Patients can present with acute on chronic urinary retention and the renal function in such cases may not recover fully. In all cases of urinary retention and renal insufficiency the patient is discharged home with indwelling catheter and any attempt at removing the catheter without definitive treatment risk further deterioration of renal function. A definitive bladder outflow surgery will be required if the patient is fit for anaesthetic. The alternative would be prostate artery embolization in selected patients, especially the elderly and frail. In some cases the interventional radiology specialist will be able to insert a suprapubic catheter at the same sitting of prostate artery embolization. The patients who undergo prostate artery embolistation will be expected to keep their indwelling catheter for several weeks after the procedure.

2.2.6   Urine Tract Infections

Many patients may present with recurrent lower urine tract infections. This may be associated with lower urinary tracts symptoms or not and occasionally patients may require hospitalisation for infection treatment in severe cases. Urine infection can be caused by stagnation from a high residual volume of urine that is not cleared after each void because of bladder outflow obstruction. Patients who require catheterisation because of retention may develop urinary infection as well. Another cause of urine infection can be the presence of bladder stones.

2.2.7   Bladder Stones

The formation of bladder stones is typically uncommon in the modern age however patients with a very large prostate are an exception and may develop primary bladder stones. Urinary stasis and high residual in addition to recurrent urine tract infection are predisposing factors. The symptoms can range from storage lower urinary tract symptoms especially dysuria and occasionally recurrent urine tract infections. Bladder stones occasionally can be asymptomatic if they are small. It is important to assess the size and the number of bladder stones as this will have implication on treatment planning. If bladder calculi are present at the time of bladder outflow surgery these can often be managed simultaneously under a single anaesthetic. If using a Greenlight PVP system or TURP then a stone punch can be utilised to crush the calculi before removal with the Ellick. If performing HoLEP then the calculi can be elegantly dusted into small fragments using the same Holmium laser. With open or robotic simple prostatectomy then the calculi can be simply lifted out. Whichever way the stones are removed it is important to minimise mucosal bleeding from sharp stone fragments which can complicate the prostate part of the surgery.

2.3 Elective Presentations

2.3.1 Elevated PSA in the Large Gland

Prostate specific antigen (PSA) level has been shown to correlate with the size of the prostate [17]. Roehrborn et al analysed more than 4600 patients from BPH trials and found PSA level and the size of the prostate are strongly inter-related. This relationship was independent of prostate cancer but was dependent on age. Older patient with larger prostates had higher PSA levels. The largest prostate volume in the trials recorded was at 70 g. This has led to the concept of PSA density which is the serum total PSA level divided by prostate volume. A value of 0.15 is generally used as the threshold level for increased suspicion of prostate cancer. Therefore, very large BPH is expected be associated with elevated PSA and in prostates over 100 cc in size it is not unusual to find a PSA level of around 10–15 ng/mL or greater, which may in fact be normal for a prostate of that size. Patients who are otherwise asymptomatic may therefore present to urologists with an elevated PSA. This usually causes one of the most difficult dilemmas in managing patients with very large BPH. In majority of the cases the moderately elevated PSA is a factor of the benign enlargement of the gland (Fig. 2.4). However, an elevation of PSA above the normal level would traditionally trigger a diagnostic process that would end with a prostate biopsy. Patients with very large prostates may be at higher risk for under-sampling of the anterior and apical regions and the prostate in general, and thus record false negative biopsy results. There is also an increased risk of significant haematuria, worsening lower urinary tract symptoms and increased rates of urinary retention post biopsies in very large glands. This dilemma is not easily solved as both large BPH and prostate cancer are common and can often co-exist. And the management should be tailored to each patient. A careful discussion should be undertaken and any decision to proceed with prostate biopsies should only be undertaken after full counselling ensuring the patient is aware of these specifically increased risks.

Fig. 2.4 (**a**) MRI of prostate—coronal view. (**b**) MRI of prostate—sagittal view. (**c**) MRI of prostate—axial view. (**a–c**) A Large prostate on a MRI scan on of a 75 year old man with LUTS, IPSS: 27/35, the volume of the prostate was calculated at 270cc. This patient underwent Holmium laser enucleation of the prostate and pre- operative PSA was 7. Post-operatively PSA: 0.69

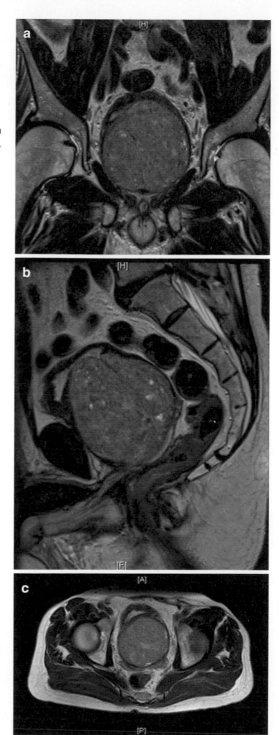

A multi- parametric MRI (1.5 or preferably 3 Tesla) with an experienced uro-radiologist can play a very helpful role in selecting which patients should go forward to prostate biopsies. As well as showing potential areas of prostate cancer, the prostate size and shape, it can also identify signs of bladder outflow obstruction such as bladder thickening, calculi, diverticula, hydronephrosis, and prostatic middle lobes. Many patients with a reassuring PSA density (<0.15 ng/mL/cc) and no obvious signs of cancer may be able to avoid biopsy. Indeed a mildly elevated PSA with a non-suspicious MRI (PIRADS score 1 or 2) can be safely followed up with regular PSA and occasional MRI without the need for prostate biopsies.

2.3.2   Incidental Imaging

Patients who are incidentally found to have a very large prostate can be referred to urology services for full lower urinary tract symptoms assessment which may include digital rectal examination, serum creatinine, urine analysis, flow rate and bladder residual in addition to urinary tract ultrasound scan. Should the patient be found not to have any bothersome symptoms with no evidence of bladder outflow obstruction then they can be safely followed up with renal function, IPSS score and regular flow rate at the primary care level.

Occasionally a bladder ultrasound scan can report a large bladder tumour erroneously which eventually is revealed to be a large middle lobe of the prostate [18].

2.3.3   Lower Urinary Tract Symptoms

Most patients with a very large prostate will experience some lower urinary tract symptoms and may present with these issues. Although many men will having primarily voiding symptoms, a high percentage of these patients will have mixed storage and voiding symptoms due to excessive voiding pressures causing secondary detrusor over-activity. In these patient often the offending element is the very large middle lobe that is intruding into the bladder. This intrusion contributes to the storage symptoms and medical therapy is usually less effective. The anatomy of the middle lobe is different from the lateral lobes of the prostate. The lateral lobes surround the prostatic urethra at the bladder neck where the effect of alpha blockers and 5-alpha reductase inhibitors would be maximal. If the clinical assessment reveals a very large prostate >100 cc then there should be a low threshold for medical or eventually surgical intervention. Although the usual pathway is to start an alpha-blocker in isolation, these men are more likely to benefit from combination therapy with a 5-alpha reductase inhibitor initiated at an early stage. This will be more likely to prevent the need for bladder outflow surgery and urinary retention. If symptoms fail to respond to medical therapy it is often due to a large middle lobe indenting into the trigone, acting like a ball-valve, and cause voiding symptoms. These patients do not usually benefit from medical therapy and are best treated with bladder outflow surgery earlier rather than later.

2.3.4 Mass Effect

This is a relatively unusual presentation. Patients can feel a continuous fullness in their rectum (tensemus) and complain of difficulty in defecation. This is due to the very large prostate filling most of the space in the pelvis in addition to the increased voiding pressures at the time of micturition. Some relief will be provided by medical therapies but there should be a low threshold for bladder outflow surgery.

2.3.5 Asymptomatic

Some patients with very large prostate may remain very well without any symptoms. In a case reported by Dominguez [7], a patient with a prostate measured at almost 4000 mL has remained asymptomatic without any signs of bladder outflow obstruction and avoided surgery. However, the patient remained under urological follow up.

2.4 Summary

- Patients with very large prostate can be asymptomatic
- Very large prostate can be mistaken for bladder cancer on imaging
- Large prostate may require special curved catheters in case of retention
- Large prostate can cause problematic recurrent haematuria which can be difficult to manage
- Blind suprapubic catheterisation is not recommended in men with very large prostates
- PSA can be elevated in very large prostate; mp-MRI and PSA density can help identify patients at risk of prostate cancer

References

1. Boyle P, Gould AL, Roehrborn CG. Prostate volume predicts outcome of treatment of benign prostatic hyperplasia with finasteride: meta-analysis of randomized clinical trials. Urology. 1996;48:398–405.
2. Cunha GR, Donjacour AA, Cooke PS, et al. The endocrinology and developmental biology of the prostate. Endocr Rev. 1987;8:338–62.
3. Timms BG, Mohs TJ, Didio LJ. Ductal budding and branching patterns in the developing prostate. J Urol. 1994;151:1427–32.
4. Wilson JD. The pathogenesis of benign prostatic hyperplasia. Am J Med. 1980;68:745–56.
5. Georgiades F, Demosthenous S, Antoniades G, Kouriefs C. Giant benign prostatic hyperplasia in a young adult male. Urology. 2014;84:e4–5.

6. Wroclawski ML, Carneiro A, Tristao RA, et al. Giant prostatic hyperplasia: report of a previously asymptomatic man presenting with gross hematuria and hypovolemic shock. Einstein (Sao Paulo). 2015;13:420–2.
7. Dominguez A, Gual J, Munoz-Rodriguez J, et al. Giant Prostatic Hyperplasia: Case Report of 3987 mL. Urology. 2016;88:e3–4.
8. Fishman JR, Merrill DC. A case of giant prostatic hyperplasia. Urology. 1993;42:336–7.
9. Jones P, Alzweri L, Rai BP, Somani BK, Bates C, Aboumarzouk OM. Holmium laser enucleation versus simple prostatectomy for treating large prostates: Results of a systematic review and meta-analysis. Arab J Urol. 2016;14:50–8.
10. Cornu JN, Ahyai S, Bachmann A, et al. A Systematic Review and Meta-analysis of Functional Outcomes and Complications Following Transurethral Procedures for Lower Urinary Tract Symptoms Resulting from Benign Prostatic Obstruction: An Update. Eur Urol. 2015;67:1066–96.
11. Bhindi B, Margel D, Trottier G, et al. Obesity is associated with larger prostate volume but not with worse urinary symptoms: analysis of a large multiethnic cohort. Urology. 2014;83:81–7.
12. He Q, Babcook MA, Shukla S, et al. Obesity-initiated metabolic syndrome promotes urinary voiding dysfunction in a mouse model. Prostate. 2016;76:964–76.
13. Patel ND, Parsons JK. Epidemiology and etiology of benign prostatic hyperplasia and bladder outlet obstruction. Indian J Urol. 2014;30:170–6.
14. He Q, Wang Z, Liu G, Daneshgari F, MacLennan GT, Gupta S. Metabolic syndrome, inflammation and lower urinary tract symptoms: possible translational links. Prostate Cancer Prostatic Dis. 2016;19:7–13.
15. Hunter DJ, Berra-Unamuno A, Martin-Gordo A. Prevalence of urinary symptoms and other urological conditions in Spanish men 50 years old or older. J Urol. 1996;155:1965–70.
16. Roehrborn CG. Accurate determination of prostate size via digital rectal examination and transrectal ultrasound. Urology. 1998;51:19–22.
17. Roehrborn CG, Boyle P, Gould AL, Waldstreicher J. Serum prostate-specific antigen as a predictor of prostate volume in men with benign prostatic hyperplasia. Urology. 1999;53:581–9.
18. Ibrahim AG, Mohammed BS, Aliyu S, Wabada S, Iya AM, Sanda AB. Giant median lobe enlargement of the prostate mimicking advanced bladder tumour: a case report. West Afr J Med. 2014;33:74–6.

Chapter 3
Imaging of the Large Prostate

Jan Philipp Radtke, Claudia Kesch, and David Bonekamp

3.1 Introduction

Prostate cancer (PCa) is the most commonly diagnosed cancer in European men (382,000 new cases annually: 22% of all male cancer cases).

Multiparametric magnetic resonance imaging (mpMRI), combining anatomic and functional imaging techniques for evaluating the prostate is increasingly being used in the diagnosis and management of PCa. With the use of mpMRI, the accuracy for the diagnosis of PCa has significantly increased in recent years, and this has already led to changes in the diagnostic pathway [1–4]. In addition, the implementation of a standardized classification system (PI-RADS) has led to more consistent reporting and aided the dissemination of mpMRI [5, 6]. A wide spectrum of anatomic and pathologic processes within the prostate may masquerade as PCa, complicating the interpretation of MRI [7]. These entities include the anterior fibromuscular stroma (AFMS), the central zone (CZ), benign prostatic hyperplasia (BPII), atrophy, necrosis, calcification, hemorrhage and prostatitis [7]. Understanding of the prostate zonal anatomy and pathophysiology is helpful to distinguish benign entities from PCa. The AFMS and CZ are characteristic anatomic features of the prostate associated with a low T2 signal intensity due to dense fibromuscular or complex crowded glandular tissue [7–9]. BPH, atrophy, necrosis, calcification, and hemorrhage all have characteristic features with one or more specific mpMRI modalities [7, 8]. It is important for both radiologists and urologists to be

J.P. Radtke (✉)
Department of Urology, University Medical Center Heidelberg, Heidelberg, Germany

Department of Radiology, German Cancer Research Center (DKFZ), Heidelberg, Germany
e-mail: j.radtke@dkfz-heidelberg.de

C. Kesch
Department of Urology, University Medical Center Heidelberg, Heidelberg, Germany
e-mail: claudia.kesch@med.uni-heidelberg.de

D. Bonekamp
Department of Radiology, German Cancer Research Center (DKFZ), Heidelberg, Germany
e-mail: d.bonekamp@dkfz-heidelberg.de

© Springer International Publishing AG 2018
V. Kasivisvanathan, B. Challacombe (eds.), *The Big Prostate*,
https://doi.org/10.1007/978-3-319-64704-3_3

familiar with specific benign imaging findings when interpreting not only prostate MR images, but also ultrasound (US). In this chapter, we focus not only on these imaging findings, but also on the correlation of MRI findings with the International Prostate Symptom Score (IPSS) and on the role of MRI in the follow-up of medical or interventional treatment of BPH.

3.2 Imaging of the Enlarged Prostate: Challenges and Suggestions

Prostate volume estimates are becoming more important because the choice of treatment is increasingly based on such estimates [10]. Digital-rectal examination (DRE) is the simplest way to assess prostate volume, but the correlation to prostate volume is poor [10, 11]. Quality-control procedures for DRE have been described [12]. Transrectal ultrasound (TRUS) is more accurate in determining prostate volume than DRE. Underestimation of prostate volume by DRE increases with increasing TRUS volume, particularly where the volume is >30 mL [13]. In routine clinical practice, methods that can accurately estimate the degree of prostatic enlargement in individuals (in contrast to the exact volume) are sufficient if one wants to avoid overtreating or undertreating a significant percentage of men [14]. However, even TRUS misses accurate exact volume estimation [15]. Imaging very enlarged prostates up to 100 mL seems challenging on TRUS and the diagnostic workflow in urology practice is unclear [16] (Fig. 3.1).

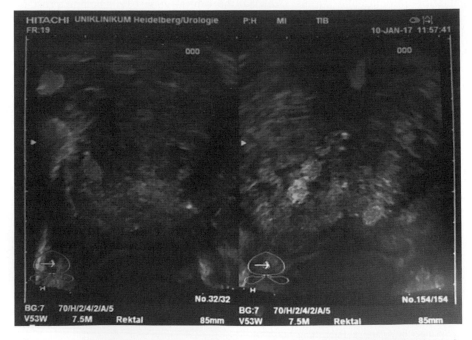

Fig. 3.1 Enlarged prostate (130 mL volume) with complete suppression of the peripheral zone in favor of the enlarged central gland. The hyperechogenic lesions are calcifications

Often an enlarged prostate is firstly diagnosed adjacently on computed tomography [17]. Because of its inferior soft tissue contrast, compared to MRI or TRUS is not considered the primary imaging method when examining the prostate [17].

Whereas Roehrborn et al. analysed that the accuracy and reproducibility of TRUS in enlarged prostates is not inferior in smaller ones, Stravodimos et al. demonstrated that the accuracy of TRUS is higher in prostates below 80 mL compared to larger ones [16, 18]. To our knowledge, only this study analyzed median prostate volumes above 100 mL [16]. They demonstrated a miscategorization rate (below or above 80 cc, derived from the EAU guideline recommendation on open or endourologic treatment for benign prostate hyperplasia) of 13% [16, 19]. However, compared to transabdominal US, the correlation of TRUS-measured volume to histopathology specimen volume was significantly higher [16]. In conclusion, TRUS could probably be considered as a standard means of evaluation for a BPH patient population [16]. One study compared MRI and TRUS in enlarged prostates, however, the median volume did not reach 100 mL (39 mL) [20]. They found a higher correlation for MRI and histopathology volume compared to TRUS [20] (Fig. 3.2).

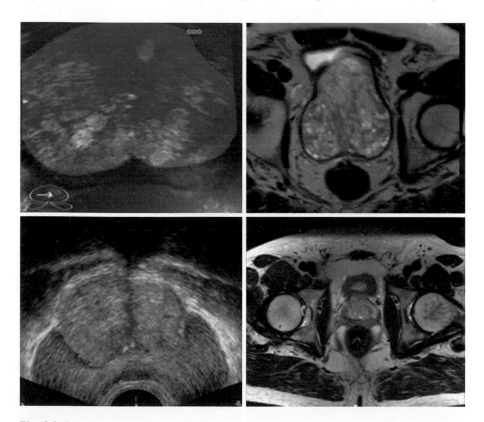

Fig. 3.2 Imaging appearances of the large prostate on US and MRI and differences between appearances of a large and small prostate. *Top left* and *top right*: an enlarged prostate in a 65-year old man with 130 mL prostate volume. *Top left*: ultrasound image demonstrating enlarged central gland (*yellow*) and compressed peripheral zone (red). *Top right*: T2-weighted MR image of the same prostate in transverse plane. Note that the compressed peripheral zone can hardly be seen. *Bottom left* and *bottom right*: regular sized 25 mL gland in a 68-year old man with enlarged central gland (*yellow*), but regular appearance of uncompressed peripheral zone (*red*); *Bottom left:* ultrasound image; *bottom right*: T2-weighted MR image in transverse plane

In addition, MRI slightly overestimated the exact volume by 1.4 mL, while TRUS underestimated it by 3.4 mL [20]. The presence of a median lobe is a significant predictor of accurate prostate volume measurement for both MRI and TRUS and may lead to volume overestimation when using the prolate ellipsoid formula [20].

Besides the volume measurement of MRI alone, the diagnostic accuracy of different modalities varies for enlarged versus smaller prostates.

Regarding PCa detection, both sensitivity and specificity of systematic TRUS guided biopsy decreased as the prostate enlarged, especially for prostates greater than 40 mL [21, 22]. Several groups reported a PCa detection rate less than 30% for prostates greater than 40 mL compared to a higher detection rate for smaller glands [22–24].

Multiparametric MRI is increasingly recognized as a method of detecting PCa, especially in men with an enlarged gland [25–27].

Publications on differences of functional imaging for BPH, especially transition zone (TZ) or CZ changes, between different prostate volumes are lacking.

However, for urologists it is important to know strengths and limitations of functional ultrasound and MR imaging and to choose the right imaging modality for their specific question. The following sections elucidate functional imaging of both ultrasound (mainly TRUS) and MRI for enlarged prostates. It is important to acknowledge that these suggestions on different modalities in specific situations are not hierarchical. TRUS has been the most common and initially applied imaging modality for prostate diseases, being available in most private practices and hospitals. Recently, new concepts are posed to improve its diagnostic efficacy even in specific functional questions. Based on an accurate size estimation using TRUS, urologists should be able to choose an appropriate imaging modality to answer their clinical question (B-plane or color-doppler US and native or functional MRI with or without contrast agent) (Fig. 3.3).

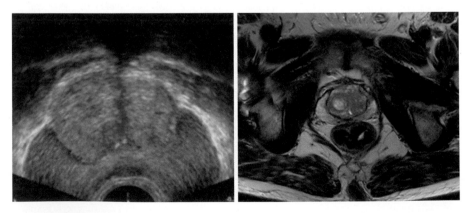

Fig. 3.3 Figure showing the zonal anatomy (*red*: peripheral zone, *yellow*: central zone) on (**a**) Ultrasound and (**b**) MR image. The transition zone is suppressed between central and peripheral zone on both images (*not colored*)

3.3   Resistive Index Measurement by Doppler

Some authors emphasized on the relationship between transitional zone index (transitional zone volume/total prostatic volume) and obstructive symptoms, mechanical bladder outlet obstruction, or acute urinary retention [28, 29]. Doppler TRUS provides information about prostate blood flow [30]. The prostate blood supply comes from urethral and capsular arteries. Enlarged transitional zone compresses the surgical capsule, so the vascular resistance in capsular artery will rise. This can be measured by Power Doppler.

Shinbo et al. studied a relationship between resistance index [(peak systolic velocity−end diastolic velocity)/peak systolic velocity], with BOO and risk of acute urinary retention in patients with BPH [29, 31]. They pointed out that resistance index with cut-off value of more than 0.75 is a more reliable predictor of BOO than international prostate symptom score (IPSS), post-void residual and transitional zone index [29, 31].

3.4   Presumed Circle Area Ratio and Capsule Elasticity

As prostate enlarges, the pressure transfers to the surgical capsule and finally at one point the capsule cannot stretch more, then prostate begins to transform to a circular shape [30]. The diversity in the elastic characteristic of surgical capsule affects this process and the final outcome will vary in different patients [30].

Presumed circle area ratio (PCAR) is calculated where the horizontal section of prostate in TRUS shows the biggest surface [30]. Then the ratio of this surface to the presumed circle with the same circumference will be calculated [30]. St Sauver et al. designed a cross-sectional study of 328 Caucasian men residing in Olmsted County, Minnesota [32]. They measured IPSS, post-void residual, peak flow rate, and PCAR. A PCAR greater than 0.9 correlates with symptom score after adjusting for age and prostate volume, but it might not provide more useful predictive information than the transitional zone volume [32].

3.5   Intraprostatic Protrusion

Intraprostatic protrusion (IPP) is mentioned as a predictive factor of obstruction in several studies. It can be performed either transabdominally or transrectally. Lee et al. investigated 256 patients with LUTS and BPH by abdominal ultrasound [33]. They measured IPP and categorized them into three subgroups: Grade 1, less than 5 mm; grade 2, 5–10 mm; and grade 3, more than 10 mm [33]. The patients received watchful waiting, alpha-blocker, or 5ARI. The authors found a relationship between a higher IPP grade and a higher risk of clinical progression regardless of the treatment types [33].

3.6 Imaging of Benign Hyperplasia: Anatomy of the Central Zone

The CZ is a layer of tissue that surrounds the ejaculatory ducts from the level of the prostatic base down to the verumontanum [10]. It is most prominent at the prostatic base and has a conical shape, with its apex at the verumontanum [10, 11]. Embryologically, the CZ originates from the Wolffian duct, whereas the TZ is a derivative of the urogenital sinus [10]. Because of its high epithelial-to-stroma ratio, the CZ accounts for 25% of the total prostate volume but almost 40% of the epithelium [34]. The CZ volume starts to decrease gradually after the age of 35 years due to reduced mean glandular activity, reduction of acinar size, and epithelial atrophy [35].

Compared to the peripheral zone, the glands of the CZ are larger and more complex, with tall columnar cells and papillary folding [35]. CZ PCa are rare, accounting for approximately 1–2% of all PCa and 3–8% of index tumors [36]. Beside their rarity, CZ PCa are usually associated with a high incidence of seminal vesicle invasion, extracapsular extension, high Gleason grade, and early biochemical failure after radical prostatectomy [36, 37] (Fig. 3.4).

On MR imaging, the normal CZ appears homogeneously hypointense on T2-weighted imaging with low ADC values on diffusion-weighted imaging (DWI) in patients between 42 and 84 years of age [7, 39, 40]. As PCa carries as similar signature, correct anatomical identification of the CZ is necessary to avoid misdi-

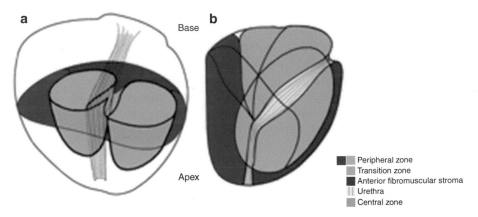

Fig. 3.4 Scheme of prostate zones: Transversal (**a**) and sagittal (**b**) scheme of prostate zones, according to McNeal et al. and adapted from Bouye et al. [10, 38]. The *dark green* colored area represents the anterior fibromuscular stroma and the *bright green* colored area the transition zone of the prostate. The peripheral zone is colored in *blue*, the normal central zone in *grey*

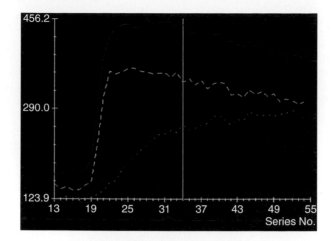

Fig. 3.5 Figure showing the three Dynamic contrast enhancement (DCE) curves: Type I, green curve—progressive enhancement. Type II, yellow curve (almost a plateau with below 20% wash-out)—rapid enhancement and plateau. Type III, red curve, rapid enhancement and washout

agnosis. Features that allow distinction of the CZ are the symmetric appearance and its typical shape and location [40]. It is important to notice that in 20% of cases the CZ may be asymmetric, increasing difficulty of assessment [40]. An enlarged TZ can lead to compression of the CZ. At DCE imaging, the CZ has been shown to be associated with type 1 (progressive) and type 2 (early enhancement and plateau phase) rather than type 3 (early enhancement and washout) enhancement curve types [7] (Fig. 3.5).

BPH is defined as enlargement of the TZ and characterized by hyperplasia of both prostatic stromal and epithelial cells, resulting in formation of large discrete nodules [35]. Histologically, BPH nodules appear as stromal or glandular proliferation or dilatation and fibromuscular proliferation of the stroma [35]. This composition results in a typical heterogeneous appearance of BPH on T2-weighted images [41].

On MRI, BPH nodules may occur as hypo-, iso-, or hyperintense on T2-weighted imaging, depending on the ratio of glandular to stromal tissue [7, 42]. Kitzing et al. stated that high signal intensity is due to hyperplastic glandular elements, which are filled with secretions, and the presence of cystic ductal ectasia [7]. Cystic/glandular BPH nodules are very often present on imaging and can be straightforwardly differentiated from PCa due to their typical imaging appearance. Stromal BPH may mimic PCa due to its low and sometimes irregular T2 signal and the presence of unsharp lesion margins without well-defined capsule (Fig. 3.6).

Fig. 3.6 BPH nodules within the central zone of the prostate gland on a T2-weighted coronar image. The BPH nodules (*white arrows*) are mild and severely hyperintense

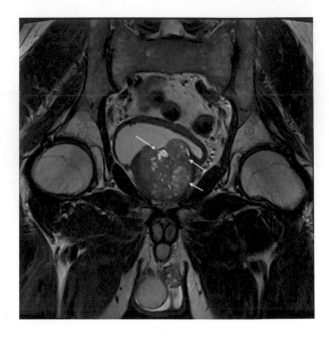

3.7   Imaging Benign Prostate Hyperplasia and Correlation of MRI and International Prostate Symptom Score (IPSS)

Traditionally, transrectal ultrasound (TRUS) has been used when imaging evaluation of BPH is required. The increased use of MRI is mainly geared toward its ability to detect, localize and grade PCa [43]. BPH is imaged on MRI most commonly as an incidental finding in patients with a clinical suspicion of PCa, a common occurrence as the BPH is the most common contributor to PSA increases apart from PCa. BPH is therefore a frequent confounder of MRI interpretation for PCa and excellent understanding of the MR imaging appearance is required for high-quality prostate MRI reporting. The study of BPH therefore furthers both, the diagnostic ability of MRI for the detection of PCa and the understanding of BPH itself. As such, MRI has been recently used to refine BPH classification. According to Wasserman et al. BPH types on MRI are defined as follows: Type 0, an equal to or less than 25 cm³ prostate showing little or no zonal enlargement, Type 1: bilateral TZ enlargement (35%), Type 2: retrourethral enlargement (10%), Type 3: bilateral TZ and retrourethral enlargement (46%), Type 4: solitary or multiple pedunculated enlargement, Type 5: pedunculated with bilateral TZ and/or retrourethral enlargement; Type 6: subtrigonal or ectopic enlargement and Type 7: other combinations of enlargements [44, 45] (Fig. 3.7).

MR imaging is not only able to depict BPH in a structured manner, but results derived from MRI can be correlated with the IPSS: Guneyli et al. analyzed the correlation of total prostate volume (TPV), TZ volume (TZV), IPP, prostatic urethra angle, bladder wall thickness, urethral changes and BPH with total IPSS in 61

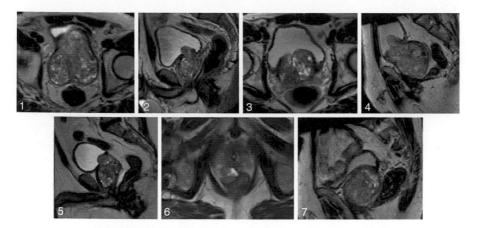

Fig. 3.7 Figure demonstrating the seven BPH types (1–7) from *top left* to *bottom right*) according to Wasserman et al. [44, 45] on MRI. *Type 1*: bilateral TZ enlargement, *Type 2*: retrourethral enlargement, *Type 3*: bilateral TZ and retrourethral enlargement, *Type 4*: solitary or multiple pedunculated enlargement, *Type 5*: pedunculated with bilateral TZ and/or retrourethral enlargement; *Type 6*: subtrigonal or ectopic enlargement and *Type 7*: other combinations of enlargements

patients. They found that TPV, TZV, IPP, AFMS changes and BPH type derived from MRI correlated significantly with IPSS [46]. In multiple linear regression analysis, TZV was the only predictor for total IPSS the scores for the IPSS questions 1 and 4 [46]. Thus, one can consider MRI findings when making treatment decisions in BPH.

3.8   Benign Pathologies That Mimic Prostate Cancer: Differentiating Benign from Malignant Lesions (Table 3.1)

Adenosis and HG-PIN are known to mimic PCa on histological evaluation [8, 34, 47]. However, these mimickers also appear to show similar characteristics on mpMRI, together with severe inflammation and with well differentiated PCa [8].

Within a mpMRI examination of the prostate high-resolution T2-WI and at least two functional MRI techniques are provided: To characterise the prostatic vascular pharmacokinetic features DCE-MRI is used. It consists of a series of axial T1-WI gradient echo sequences during and after i.v. bolus injection of gadolinium based contrast medium. Diffusion weighted imaging (DWI) with different b-values reflecting the strength and timing of the gradient used to generate the images measures the motion of water molecules within a voxel of tissue which then can be quantified in apparent diffusion coefficient (ADC) maps.

Adenosis, HG-PIN, severe inflammation and well differentiated PCa may all occur as homogenous isointense or hypointense lesions on T2-WI, usually multifocal, with moderate to low ADC values and moderate SI on high-b-value images [8]. In addition, all may show contrast enhancement with a plateau shape of the DCE curve (Type II curve) and with peak enhancement higher than that of normal glands [8].

Table 3.1 Benign pathologies that mimic prostate cancer

Potential non-malignant characteristics that mimic cancer	What it could be	Potential differentiation and difficulties
Multifocal isointense lesions with moderate low ADC value	High-grade PIN, BPH, adenosis, inflammation or PCa	High-grade PIN usually pinpoint-sized, PCa with lower ADC value; differentiation between well differentiated PCa, inflammation and adenosis very difficult
Multifocal hypointense lesion with moderate ADC value	High-grade PIN, BPH, adenosis, inflammation or PCa	High-grade PIN usually pinpoint-sized, PCa with lower ADC value; differentiation between well differentiated PCa, inflammation and adenosis very difficult
Moderate ADC value and restricted diffusion	BPH nodule, PCa, inflammation	PCa with lower ADC values, BPH nodules typically located in the transition or central zone, PCa in the peripheral zone
Low signal intensity in anterior fibromuscular stroma	Regular AFMS, PCa, fibromuscular hyperplasia	Regular AFMS with no diffusion restriction, fibromuscular hyperplasia sharply demarcated lesions, PCa with lower values on ADC
Hypointense round nodule in TZ	BPH, fibromuscular hyperplasia, PCa	BPH and fibromuscular hyperplasia sharply demarcated lesions, PCa with lower values on ADC

De Visschere et al. published that high-grade prostatic intraepithelial neoplasia (PIN) HG-PIN was found in some cases histologically [8]. However, these high-grade PINs were usually pinpoint-sized and nearly impossible to recognize on mpMRI, unless they were contrasted by surrounding structures with remarkably different signal intensities (SI) [8, 48]. On DWI, a considerable overlap in ADC values between inflammation and PCa has been reported, although ADC values are generally lower in case of PCa. The restricted diffusion in (peri)glandular inflammation may be explained by the high density of inflammatory cells [8, 49]. In the mpMRI PI-RADS scoring system such lesions are assigned a Likert score of 3, indicating that the presence of a clinically significant PCa is indeterminate [6, 50]. Poorly differentiated cancers are usually easier to discriminate from benign lesions, in particular if they present as compact and dense lesions located in the peripheral zone [47, 51]. AFMS and fibromuscular hyperplasia show similar very low SI and may act as confounders of poorly differentiated PCa on T2-weighted imaging [52, 53]. The AFMS is characterised as a crescent or spindle-shaped structure covering the prostate anteriorly [54]. Fibromuscular hyperplasia as part of BPH may occur in the TZ on T2-weighted imaging as a markedly hypointense round nodule, sharply demarcated with bulging towards the surrounding tissue [8]. Thus, DWI may be helpful in doubtful cases [8]. On DWI, poorly differentiated PCa, fibromuscular stroma and fibromuscular hyperplasia all occur with low ADC values, but on high-b-value imaging fibromuscular stroma and hyperplasia show moderate SI, whereas poorly differentiated PCa shows high SI, allowing differentiation of these lesions in many cases [8].

Overall, in areas with indistinct low SI on T2-weighted imaging, slightly decreased ADC value, contrast enhancement and slightly decreased citrate peaks it is virtually impossible to discriminate a benign lesion from well-differentiated cancer, but poorly differentiated cancers can be usually detected even in an enlarged prostate [49] (Fig. 3.8).

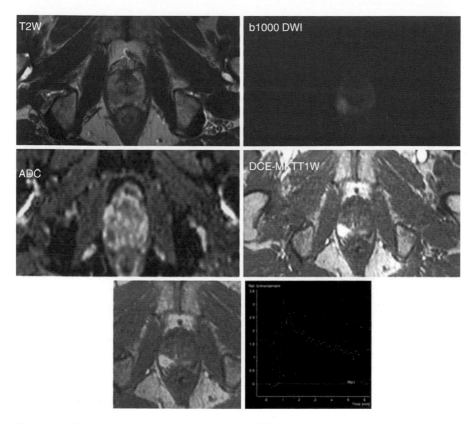

Fig. 3.8 A 68-year old man presented with a serum PSA-level of 15.6 ng/mL and a prostate volume of 87 mL. One year before, the serum PSA-level was 5.5 ng/mL. Imaging Findings: In the right mid PZpm/pl, T2W imaging detected a large hypointense lesion with capsule contact (PIRADS 5). On DWI, this lesion showed a high-signal intensity (b-value 1000 s/mm²) with a correlating low-signal-intensity on ADC map (PIRADS 5). DCE Imaging detected a positive Type III curve (PIRADS 5). Furthermore, stage T3 disease was found on T2W imaging. A second lesion was found in the left mid PZpl/pm (PIRADS 4). ADC map showed low-signal-intensity with a diffuse high-signal-intensity focus on DWI (b-value 1000 s/mm²). DCE Imaging detected a Type I curve (not shown). 27 core-biopsy was performed. Two targeted biopsies were taken from the suspicious area in the right mid PZpm/pl and one from the left mid PZpl/pm. 24 systematic cores were taken according to the Ginsburg Study Group Scheme. A prostate cancer Gleason Score 4 + 5 was found in the two targeted cores of the right mid PZpm/pl and in the systematic biopsy cores on the right. A Gleason Score 3 + 3 tumour was found in the systematic cores biopsies from the left mid PZpl/pm. A classical radical prostatectomy was performed. Histopathological examination detected a pT3b pN0 (0/19) R0 Gleason Score 4 + 5 prostate cancer on the right. The tumour volume was 4.0 mL

3.9   5-Alpha Reductase Blockade, Alpha-1 Antagonists and Prostatic Artery Embolization: Monitoring Using MRI

MRI is not only a reliable tool for the diagnosis of BPH and its distinction from PCa, it may also be used to evaluate the efficacy of BPH treatment, such as 5-alpha reductase blockade and prostatic artery embolization (PAE).

In a canine model, Jia et al. demonstrated that DCE, and in particular the pharmacokinetic maximum enhancement ratio (MER) correlated with decreased parenchyma after finasteride treatment [55]. In their study, the therapy-induced prostate volume changes under finasteride treatment were assessed [55]. The changes in prostate volume at the end of the trial exhibited a significant linear correlation to the initial parenchymal MER (p = 0.02) in the finasteride group [55]. The authors conclude that the parenchymal MER in DCE-MRI exhibits a significant linear relationship to the change in prostate volume and that these findings show great promise in using the pharmacokinetic parameter as a predictor of subject response to 5a-reductase inhibitors [55]. In contrast to the previous results, Isen et al. analyzed if clinical outcome after terazosin treatment can be measured using MRI and found no statistically significant relationship between the clinical outcome of terazosin and the MRI findings [56].

PAE is a minimally invasive therapy that has been shown to be safe and effective for relief from LUTS associated with BPH [57, 58].

Several publications analyzed the utility of MRI in the follow-up and monitoring after PAE. Frenk et al. analyzed a cohort of 17 men following PAE for a follow-up period of 18 months [59]. They stated that prostatic infarcts were seen in 71% of patients, exclusively in the central gland, and that these were almost always characterized by hyperintensity on T1-weighted images and predominant hypointensity on T2-weighted images. Volume reduction of the prostate on MRI after PAE was significant (average 32% after 12–18 months; p < 0.001) only in patients with infarcts [59]. MRI was not only used in the intermediate- and long-term follow-up, but also to analyze PAE outcome in the early post-treatment phase. Kisilevzky et al. analyzed a cohort of 24 men after PAE [60]. Prostate volume decreased 24% in successfully treated patients versus 16% (p = 0.03) in the unsuccessful cases [60]. The presence of ischemia on postoperative MRI and the MRI-measured volume were significant predictors of a successful PAE on multivariate analysis [60].

To summarize, parenchymal MER in DCE-MRI might be a valuable predictor of patient response to 5a-reductase inhibitors but so far no other MRI parameters have been found predicting or monitoring patients clinical outcome according to IPSS after BPH treatment with 5a-reductase inhibitors or PAE.

3.10   MRI, TRUS and MRI/TRUS-Fusion Biopsies in Enlarged Prostates: Are There Any Differences Compared to Smaller Organs?

Initial studies to investigate differences in diagnostic accuracy between regular and enlarged prostates were performed with prostate volume as primary endpoint [18, 61]. Both publications analyzed the correlation coefficients for inter-reader reproducibility of TRUS-measured prostate volumes [18, 61]. The correlation coefficients ranged from 0.61 to 0.72 for three examiners [18]. Total prostate volume reproducibility was higher for prostate volume greater than 40 mL compared to smaller prostates [61]. Regarding PCa detection, both sensitivity and specificity of systematic TRUS guided biopsy decreased as the prostate enlarged, especially for prostates greater than 40 mL [21, 22]. Several groups reported a PCa detection rate less than 30% for prostates greater than 40 mL compared to a higher detection rate for smaller glands [22–24]. Most authors hypothesize that this is related to sampling error since core biopsies are obtained randomly in the prostate gland and lesions are often small, heterogeneous and not uniformly distributed [27, 62]. In addition it is proposed that the increased amount of glandular tissue in larger prostates increases the potential of harboring more PCa [27]. When a standardized number of biopsy cores is taken, larger prostates may possibly predispose to undersampling [27]. Thus, in men with BPH PCa may remain undiagnosed for longer periods of time [27]. These patients commonly undergo multiple biopsy attempts, extended or even saturation biopsies with the resultant increased risk of procedure related complications [62]. Multiparametric MRI is increasingly recognized as a method of detecting PCa, especially in men with an enlarged gland [25, 26, 63, 64].

The detection rate of TRUS guided biopsy for prostate glands greater than 40 mL is considerably lower than for glands smaller than 40 mL [27]. A detection rate ranging from 40% in glands less than 34 mL to 24% in glands greater than 64 mL was reported by Ung et al. in a cohort of 750 consecutive patients with a median prostate volume of 45 mL [22]. Yoon et al. similarly noted a yield ranging from 30% in glands less than 40 mL to 27% for a prostate volume of 40 mL or greater in a cohort of 474 patients [24]. Even when performing 20-core TRUS guided biopsy, Werahera et al. reported a 26% PCa detection rate in men with a prostate of greater than 50 mL [23]. However, when using MRI/TRUS-fusion biopsies, Walton-Diaz et al. demonstrated a higher PCa detection rate of 48% for glands of 40 mL or greater compared to the previous TRUS controls using MRI/TRUS-fusion biopsies [27]. They added that the detection rate of high-risk PCa using MR/TRUS-fusion did not decrease with enlarged prostate volume [27]. In addition, the authors demonstrated that MRI/TRUS-fusion biopsies showed superior PCa detection compared to extended sextant TRUS guided biopsy [27]. Also, de Gorski et al. analyzed the utility of MRI/TRUS-fusion biopsies compared to 12-core standard TRUS biopsies for the detection of PCa in enlarged prostates (greater 40 mL) in a cohort of 232 men [65]. They found that differences in prostate cancer detection rates between the standard and targeted protocols were not significant for patients with a prostate volume of 40 mL or less (p = 0.8) [65]. Conversely 12 patients with a prostate volume greater than 40 mL had clinically significant PCa using the targeted but not the standard protocol and in 3 PCa was detected by the standard but not the targeted protocol (p = 0.04) [65]. They conclude that in prostates greater than 40 mL, it may be necessary to systematically perform MRI/TRUS-fusion biopsies rather than systematic biopsies as a first line approach to ensure accurate diagnosis [65].

Particularly in the enlarged prostate, MRI/TRUS-fusion biopsies may offer many advantages when compared to conventional TRUS guided biopsy, but the ideal protocol is still yet to be established.

3.11   Conclusion

When patients with enlarged prostates present, the initial imaging modality might be transabdominal US or TRUS. TRUS accurately examines the prostate volume. Furthermore, it can provide information on the blood flow, measured by resistive index, which can be, in case of an increased resistive index, a surrogate of an enlarged TZ. Also the PCAR can be derived from TRUS and correlates well with the IPSS. Lastly, IPP, measured by US, correlates well with the clinical progression risk of BPH. In the evaluation of patients with clinical symptoms or unclear PSA elevation, TRUS provides important and accurate information about prostate volume, allowing to put clinical and PSA findings into context and calculate PSA density.

For further detail or to distinguish between benign and malignant findings and for treatment follow-up, MRI is a useful modality. On MR imaging the normal CZ appears homogeneously hypointense on T2-weighted imaging and with low ADC values on diffusion-weighted imaging (DWI) and should be distinguished from PCa by its typical location and morphology. BPH often demonstrates typical hypo-, iso-, or hyperintense nodules on T2-weighted imaging, however irregular margins and low T2 signal may represent diagnostic challenges especially for stromal BPH. Furthermore, adenosis and HG-PIN are known PCa mimickers on MRI and their accurate differentiation from PCa is not always possible due to an overlap in MR imaging characteristics. After treatment of benign prostate hyperplasia, MRI can be used as a reliable tool for follow-up, demonstrating typical imaging findings such as prostatic infarcts. Quantitative color-imaged morphometric analysis on MRI has shown ability to predict positive IPSS outcome after 5-alpha reductase blockade.

In case of remaining PCa suspicion, the very large prostate in particular should be investigated using mpMRI, with the option for further targeted biopsies to allow for an accurate diagnosis, rather than performing standard TRUS biopsy or saturation TRUS biopsy.

References

1. Siddiqui MM, Rais-Bahrami S, Turkbey B, George AK, Rothwax J, Shakir N, et al. Comparison of MR/ultrasound fusion-guided biopsy with ultrasound-guided biopsy for the diagnosis of prostate cancer. JAMA. 2015;313(4):390. http://jama.jamanetwork.com/article.aspx?doi=10.1001/jama.2014.17942
2. Baco E, Ukimura O, Rud E, Vlatkovic L, Svindland A, Aron M, et al. Magnetic resonance imaging – transectal ultrasound image-fusion biopsies accurately characterize the index tumor : correlation with step-sectioned radical prostatectomy specimens in 135 patients. Eur Urol. 2015;67(4):787–94.
3. Radtke JP, Schwab C, Wolf MB, Freitag MT, Alt CD, Kesch C, et al. Multiparametric magnetic resonance imaging (MRI) and MRI–transrectal ultrasound fusion biopsy for index tumor detection: correlation with radical prostatectomy specimen. Eur Urol. 2016;pii: S0302(16):00010–5. http://dx.doi.org/10.1016/j.eururo.2015.12.052
4. Ahmed HU, El-Shater Bosaily A, Brown L, Kaplan RS, Colaco-Moraes Y, Ward K, et al. PROMIS study: Diagnostic accuracy of multi-parametric MRI and TRUS biopsy in prostate cancer (PROMIS): a paired validating confirmatory study. The Lancet 2017;6736(16):32401–1.
5. Barentsz JO, Richenberg J, Clements R, Choyke P, Verma S, Villeirs G, et al. ESUR prostate MR guidelines 2012. Eur Radiol. 2012;22:746–57.
6. Weinreb JC, Barentsz JO, Choyke PL, Cornud F, Haider MA, Macura KJ, et al. PI-RADS prostate imaging-Reporting and data system 2015, version 2. Eur Urol. 2016;69:16–40. doi: 10.1016/j.eururo.2015.08.052
7. Kitzing YX, Prando A, Varol C, Karczmar GS, Maclean F, Oto A. Benign conditions that mimic prostate carcinoma: MR imaging features with histopathologic. Radiographics. 2016;36:162–75.
8. De Visschere PJL, Vral A, Perletti G, Pattyn E, Praet M, Magri V, et al. Multiparametric magnetic resonance imaging characteristics of normal, benign and malignant conditions in the prostate. Eur Radiol. 2017;27(5):2095-2109. http://dx.doi.org/10.1007/s00330-016-4479-z
9. Li Y, Mongan J, Behr S, Sud S, Coakley F V, Simko JP, et al. Beyond prostate adenocarcinoma: expanding the differential diagnosis in prostate pathologic conditions. Radiographics. 2016;(36):1055–1075.
10. McNeal JE. The zonal anatomy of the prostate. Prostate. 1981;2:35–49.
11. Fine SW, Reuter VE. Anatomy of the prostate revisited: implications for prostate biopsy and zonal origins of prostate cancer. Histopathology. 2012;60(1):142–52. http://www.ncbi.nlm.nih.gov/pubmed/22212083
12. Weissfeld JL, Fagerstrom RM, O'Brien B, Prostate, Lung C; OCSTPT. Quality control of cancer screening examination procedures in the Prostate, Lung, Colorectal and Ovarian (PLCO) Cancer Screening Trial. Control Clin Trials. 2000;21(6 Suppl):390S–399S.
13. Roehrborn CG. Accurate determination of prostate size via digital rectal examination and transrectal ultrasound. Urology. 1998;51(4A Suppl):19–22.
14. Bosch JLHR, Bohnen AM, Groeneveld FPMJ. Validity of digital rectal examination and serum prostate specific antigen in the estimation of prostate volume in community-based men aged 50 to 78 years: The Krimpen Study. Eur Urol. 2004;46:753–9.
15. Nathan MS, Seenivasagam K, Mei Q, Wickham JE, Miller JE. Transrectal ultrasonography: Why are estimates of prostate volume and dimension so inaccurate? Br J Urol. 1996;77:401–407.

16. Stravodimos KG, Petrolekas A, Kapetanakis T, Vourekas S, Koritsiadis G, Adamakis I, et al. TRUS versus transabdominal ultrasound as a predictor of enucleated adenoma weight in patients with BPH. Int Urol Nephrol. 2009;41:767–71.

17. Gossner J. Computed tomography of the prostate—a review. Int J Radiol. 2012;14(1):1–7.

18. Roehrborn CG, Sech S, Montoya J, Rhodes T, Girman CJ. Interexaminer reliability and validity of a three-dimensional model to assess prostate volume by digital rectal examination. Urology. 2001;57(6):1087–92.

19. Gratzke C, Bachmann A, Descazeaud A, Drake MJ, Madersbacher S, Mamoulakis C, et al. EAU guidelines on the assessment of non-neurogenic male lower urinary tract symptoms including benign prostatic obstruction. Eur Urol. 2015;67(6):1099–109.

20. Paterson NR, Lavallée LT, Nguyen LN, Witiuk K, Ross J, Mallick R, et al. Prostate volume estimations using magnetic resonance imaging and transrectal ultrasound compared to radical prostatectomy specimens. Can Urol Assoc J. 2016;10(7–8):264–8.

21. Karakiewicz PI, Bazinet M, Aprikian AG, Trudel C, Aronson S, Nachabe M, et al. Outcome of sextant biopsy according to gland volume. Urology. 1997;49(1):55–9.

22. Ung JO, San Francisco IF, Regan MM, Dewolf WC, Olumni AF. The relationship of prostate gland volume to extended needle biopsy on prostate cancer detection. J Urol. 2003;169(1):130–5.

23. Werahera PN, Sullivan K, La Rosa FG, Kim FJ, Lucia MS, O'Donnell C, et al. Optimization of prostate cancer diagnosis by increasing the number of core biopsies based on gland volume. Int J Clin Exp Pathol. 2012;5(9):892–9.

24. Yoon BI, Shin TS, Cho HJ, Hong SH, Lee JY, Hwang TK, et al. Is it effective to perform two more prostate biopsies according to prostate-specific antigen level and prostate volume in detecting prostate cancer? Prospective study of 10-core and 12-core prostate biopsy. Urol J. 2012;9(2):491–7.

25. Natarajan S, Marks LS, Margolis DJ, Huang J, Macairan M, Lieu P, et al. Clinical application of a 3D ultrasound-guided prostate biopsy system. Urol Oncol. 2011;29(3):334–42.

26. Singh AK, Kruecker J, Xu S, Glossop ND, Guion P, Ullman K, et al. Initial clinical experience with real-time transrectal ultrasonography-magnetic resonance imaging fusion-guided prostate biopsy. BJU Int. 2008;101(7):841–5.

27. Walton Diaz A, Hoang AN, Turkbey B, Hong CW, Truong H, Sterling T, et al. Can magnetic resonance-ultrasound fusion biopsy improve cancer detection in enlarged prostates? J Urol. 2013;190(6):2020–5. http://www.ncbi.nlm.nih.gov/pubmed/23792130

28. Kurita Y, Masuda H, Terada H, Suzuki K, Fujita K. Transition zone index as a risk factor for acute urinary retention in benign prostatic hyperplasia. Urology. 1998;51(4):595–600.

29. Shinbo H, Kurita Y. Application of ultrasonography and the resistive index for evaluating bladder outlet obstruction in patients with benign prostatic hyperplasia. Curr Urol Rep. 2011;12(4):255–60.

30. Abdi H, Kazzazi A, Bazargani ST, Djavan B. Imaging in benign prostatic hyperplasia: what is new? Curr Opin Urol 2013;23:11–16.

31. Shinbo H, Kurita Y, Takada S, Imanishi T, Otsuka A, Furuse H, et al. Resistive index as risk factor for acute urinary retention in patients with benign prostatic hyperplasia. Urology. 2010;76(6):1440–5.

32. St Stauver JL, Jacobson DJ, McGree ME, Girman CJ, Nehra A, Lieber MM, et al. Presumed circle area ratio of the prostate in a community-based group of men. BJU Int. 2009;104(1):58–62.

33. Lee LS, Sim HG, Lim K Bin, Wang D, Foo KT. Intravesical prostatic protrusion predicts clinical progression of benign prostatic enlargement in patients receiving medical treatment. Int J Urol 2010;17:69–74.

34. McNeal JE. Normal histology of the prostate. Am J Surg Pathol. 1988;12(8):619–33.

35. McNeal JE. McNeal JE; Burroughs Wellcome C. The prostate gland: morphology and pathobiology. In: The prostate gland: morphology and pathobiology. Princeton: Burroughs Wellcome. 1983.

36. Cohen RJ, Shannon BA, Phillips M, Moorin RE, Wheeler TM, Garrett K. Central zone carcinoma of the prostate gland: a distinct tumor type with poor prognostic features. J Urol. 2008;179(5):1762–7.
37. Noguchi M, Stamey TA, Neal JE, Yemoto CE. An analysis of 148 consecutive transition zone cancers: clinical and histological characteristics. J Urol. 2000;163:1751–5.
38. Bouye S, Potiron E, Puech P, Leroy X, Lemaitre L, Villers A. Transition zone and anterior stromal prostate cancers: zone of origin and intraprostatic patterns of spread at histopathology. Prostate. 2009;69(1):105–13. http://www.ncbi.nlm.nih.gov/pubmed/18850578
39. Hansford BG, Karademir I, Peng Y, Jiang Y, Karczmar G, Thomas S, et al. Dynamic contrast-enhanced MR imaging features of the normal central zone of the prostate. Acad Radiol. 2014;21(5):569–77.
40. Vargas HA, Akin O, Franiel T, Goldman DA, Udo K, Touijer KA, et al. Normal central zone of the prostate and central zone involvement by prostate cancer: clinical and MR imaging implications. Radiology. 2012;262(3):894–902.
41. Chesnais AL, Niaf E, Bratan F, Mege-Lechevallier F, Roche S, Rabilloud M, et al. Differentiation of transitional zone prostate cancer from benign hyperplasia nodules: evaluation of discriminant criteria at multiparametric MRI. Clin Radiol. 2013;68(6):e323–30. http://www.ncbi.nlm.nih.gov/pubmed/23528164
42. Hoeks CM, Hambrock T, Yakar D, Hulsbergen-van de Kaa CA, Feuth T, Witjes JA, et al. Transition zone prostate cancer: detection and localization with 3-T multiparametric MR imaging. Radiology. 2013;266(1):207–17. http://www.ncbi.nlm.nih.gov/pubmed/23143029
43. Grossfeld GD, Coakley FV. Benign prostatic hyperplasia: clinical overview and value of diagnostic imaging. Radiol Clin North Am. 2000;38(1):31–47.
44. Wasserman N. Benign prostatic hyperplasia: a review and ultrasound classification. Radiol Clin North Am. 2006;44:689–710.
45. Wasserman N, Spilseth B, Golzarian J, GJ M. Use of MRI for lobar classification of benign prostatic hyperplasia: potential phenotypic biomarkers for research on treatment strategies. AJR Am J Roentgenol. 2015;205:564–71.
46. Guneyli S, Ward E, Thomas S, Yousuf A, Trilisky I, Peng Y, et al. Magnetic resonance imaging of benign prostatic hyperplasia. Diagn Interv Radiol. 2016;22:215–9.
47. Bratan F, Niaf E, Melodelima C, Chesnais AL, Souchon R, Mege-Lechevallier F, et al. Influence of imaging and histological factors on prostate cancer detection and localisation on multiparametric MRI: a prospective study. Eur Radiol. 2013;23(7):2019–29. http://www.ncbi.nlm.nih.gov/pubmed/23494494
48. Sciarra A, Panebianco V, Ciccariello M, Salciccia S, Lisi D, Osimani M, et al. Magnetic resonance spectroscopic imaging (1H-MRSI) and dynamic contrast-enhanced magnetic resonance (DCE-MRI): pattern changes from inflammation to prostate cancer. Cancer Investig. 2010;28(4):424–32.
49. Nagel KN, Schouten MG, Hambrock T, Litjens GJ, Hoeks CM, ten Haken B, et al. Differentiation of prostatitis and prostate cancer by using diffusion-weighted MR imaging and MR-guided biopsy at 3 T. Radiology. 2013;267:164–72.
50. Barentsz JO, Richenberg J, Clements R, Choyke P, Verma S, Villeirs G, et al. ESUR prostate MR guidelines 2012. Eur Radiol. 2012;22(4):746–57. http://www.ncbi.nlm.nih.gov/pubmed/22322308
51. Rosenkrantz AB, Mendrinos S, Babb JS, Taneja SS. Prostate cancer foci detected on multiparametric magnetic resonance imaging are histologically distinct from those not detected. J Urol. 2012;187(43):2032–8.
52. Schiebler M, Schnall MD, Pollack HM, Lenkinski R, Tomaszewski JE, Wein AJ, et al. Current role of MR imaging in the staging of adenocarcinoma of the prostate. Radiology. 1993;189(2):339–352.
53. Lovett K, Rifkin M, McCue P, Choi H. MR imaging characteristics of noncancerous lesions of the prostate. J Magn Reson Imaging. 1992;2(17):35–9.

54. Coakley FV, Hricak H. Radiologic anatomy of the prostate gland: a clinical approach. Radiol Clin North Am. 2000;38(33):15–30.
55. Jia G, Heverhagen JT, Henry H, Polzer H, Baudendistel KT, von Tengg-Kobligk H, et al. Pharmacokinetic parameters as a potential predictor of response to pharmacotherapy in benign prostatic hyperplasia: a preclinical trial using dynamic contrast-enhanced MRI. Magn Reson Imaging. 2006;24(6):721–5.
56. Isen K, Sinik Z, Alkibay T, Sezer C, Sözen C, Atilla S, et al. Magnetic resonance imaging and morphometric histologic analysis of prostate tissue composition in predicting the clinical outcome of terazosin therapy in benign prostatic hyperplasia. Int J Urol. 2001;8(2):42–8.
57. Bilhim T, Pisco J, Pereira JA, Costa NV, Fernandes L, Campos Pinheiro L, et al. Predictors of clinical outcome after prostate artery embolization with spherical and nonspherical polyvinyl alcohol particles in patients with benign prostatic hyperplasia. Radiology. 2016;281(1):289–300.
58. Bagla S, Martin CP, van Breda A, Sheridan MJ, Sterling KM, Papadouris D, et al. Early results from a United States trial of prostatic artery embolization in the treatment of benign prostatic hyperplasia. J Vasc Interv Radiol. 2014;25(1):47–52.
59. Frenk NE, Carnevale FC, Antunes AA, Srougi M, Cerri GG, Ne F, et al. Artery embolization for treatment of benign hyperplasia. Am J Roentgenol. 2013;2014:813–21.
60. Kisilevzky N, Faintuch S. MRI assessment of prostatic ischaemia: best predictor of clinical success after prostatic artery embolisation for benign prostatic hyperplasia. Clin Radiol. 2016;71(9):876–882. http://dx.doi.org/10.1016/j.crad.2016.05.003
61. Sech S, Montoya J, Girman CJ, Rhodes T, Roerhborn CG. Interexaminer reliability of transrectal ultrasound for estimating prostate volume. J Urol. 2001;166(1):125–9.
62. de la Taille A, Antiphon P, Salomon L, Cherfan M, Porcher R, Hoznek A, et al. Prospective evaluation of a 21-sample needle biopsy procedure designed to improve the prostate cancer detection rate. Urology. 2003;61(6):1181–6.
63. Dickinson L, Ahmed HU, Allen C, Barentsz JO, Carey B, Futterer JJ, et al. Magnetic resonance imaging for the detection, localisation, and characterisation of prostate cancer: recommendations from a European consensus meeting. Eur Urol. 2011;59(4):477–94. http://www.ncbi.nlm.nih.gov/pubmed/21195536
64. Isebaert S, Van den Bergh L, Haustermans K, Joniau S, Lerut E, De Wever L, et al. Multiparametric MRI for prostate cancer localization in correlation to whole-mount histopathology. J Magn Reson Imaging. 2013;37(6):1392–401. http://www.ncbi.nlm.nih.gov/pubmed/23172614
65. De Gorski A, Roupret M, Peyronnet B, Le Cossec C, Granger B, Comperat E, et al. Accuracy of magnetic resonance imaging/ultrasound fusion targeted biopsies to diagnose clinically significant prostate cancer in enlarged compared to smaller prostates. J Urol. 2015;194(3):669–73.

Chapter 4
Management of an Elevated PSA and Biopsy Strategies in the Large Prostate

Joana B. Neves, Mark Emberton, and Veeru Kasivisvanathan

4.1 Large Prostates and Elevated PSA

Prostate-specific antigen (PSA) is a glycoproteic enzyme produced almost exclusively by the prostate. PSA is secreted into prostatic gland ducts and is responsible for hydrolysing the seminal clot, enabling sperm motility. In physiological conditions, only a small amount of PSA reaches intravascular circulation [1]. However, serum PSA levels can increase due to a rise in PSA production, an increase in vascular permeability, or due to disruption of tissue architecture. Thus, both benign and malignant prostatic diseases, such as benign prostatic hyperplasia (BPH), prostatitis, and prostate cancer, can be associated with increased PSA serum levels [1–3].

In a large proportion of men, aging is associated with hyperplasia of the stromal and glandular components of the transition zone leading to prostatic enlargement, also known as BPH [4–6]. Men with BPH not only have a higher baseline serum PSA before 50 years old, but are also more likely to see it increase over time [2, 7–9]. Additionally, BPH and higher prostate volumes correlate with the presence of prostate inflammation [10], a factor known to also lead to increased serum PSA readings [3].

A high serum PSA (e.g. above 3 ng/mL) is still the most frequent trigger for men to enter a suspected prostate cancer diagnostic pathway. Thus, if BPH is associated with increased PSA levels, a significant proportion of men with large prostates will be lead to have additional diagnostic tests, such as a prostate multiparametric MRI (mpMRI) and/or prostate biopsy. This represents a source of anxiety for those men as well as a burden for health care systems. However, to complicate

J.B. Neves (✉)
Division of Surgery and Interventional Science, University College London, London, UK
e-mail: joana.b.neves@ucl.ac.uk

M. Emberton • V. Kasivisvanathan
Division of Surgery and Interventional Science, University College London, London, UK

Department of Urology, University College London, London, UK
e-mail: m.emberton@ucl.ac.uk; veeru.kasi@ucl.ac.uk

© Springer International Publishing AG 2018
V. Kasivisvanathan, B. Challacombe (eds.), *The Big Prostate*,
https://doi.org/10.1007/978-3-319-64704-3_4

things further, relying solely on prostate volume to deny further diagnostic testing may be unwise as BPH and prostate cancer can co-exist and large-scale epidemiologic studies have shown that men with BPH may even be more likely to have prostate cancer [11]. Consequently, to achieve a balance between appropriate testing to identify clinically significant cancer and unnecessary testing which can lead directly and indirectly to harm, PSA readings need to be put into context and prostate volume is one of the factors to take into account.

Aiming to correctly distinguish between BPH and prostate cancer in men with elevated serum PSA, urologists and researchers have studied a number of PSA derivatives that incorporate prostate volume, such as PSA density or PSA transition zone density, have analysed PSA trends over time (PSA kinetics), have looked at different PSA isoforms, such as free PSA, and have incorporated a multitude of clinical factors, including prostate volume, into risk stratification tools. A closer look at all of these variables is warranted to assess how they can benefit clinical decision making in men with large prostates.

4.1.1 PSA Density and PSA Transition Zone Density in Large Prostates

Early studies suggest that BPH is associated with lower levels of serum PSA per volume unit of prostate than cancer (0.3 ng/mL/cc versus 3.5 ng/mL/cc) [12]. While increased serum PSA in BPH is associated with prostatic growth and higher PSA production, in prostate cancer this is thought to primarily relate to disruption of tissue architecture (namely the basal cell layer) rather than to changes in PSA production [1]. Thus, it was hypothesised that the quotient between total serum PSA and prostate volume, known as PSA density, and the quotient between total serum PSA and prostatic transition zone volume, known as PSA transition zone density, could be useful tools to discriminate men with high PSA readings who need further investigations for suspected prostate cancer from those who could avoid it.

In the early 1990s, studies based on transrectal ultrasound (TRUS) prostate volume assessment set a threshold of PSA density above 0.15 to advise men with serum PSA between 4 and 20 ng/mL to have a prostate biopsy [13, 14]. Likewise, it has been suggested that in men with raised PSA (up to 10 ng/mL), even if it is above the age-adjusted cut-off levels, a PSA density below 0.15 can lead to avoidance of unnecessary prostate biopsies [15]. However, the utility of PSA density has been undermined by further reports stating that this threshold is inadequate [16] or may only be valid for men with prostate volumes below 35 cc [17], that PSA density increases with age [2], and that in men with prostatic inflammation, a feature very commonly associated with BPH [10], PSA density may also be higher [3, 18]. Similarly, while some studies have proposed that PSA transition zone density has a better predictive value than PSA density alone [19–22], others have not confirmed this [23–25].

To date, neither PSA density nor PSA transition zone density have translated into routine clinical practice or clinical guidelines to definitively distinguish men with BPH from men with prostate cancer. However, they can be useful to make management decisions when considered alongside a full clinical picture.

Many studies looking at PSA density and PSA transition zone density have excluded men with PSA levels above 10 ng/mL. As men with very large prostates (>100 cc) are more likely to have serum PSA values well above the 3 ng/mL threshold and often at or above 10 ng/mL, the ability to draw conclusions on the role of these derivatives in the very large prostate is limited.

Nevertheless, with the increasing use of prostate mpMRI, the two biomarkers may see a resurgence since PSA levels interpreted adjusting for MRI volume information appear to improve the diagnosis of high grade prostate cancer [26] and PSA density seems to increase the diagnostic accuracy of MRI when images are equivocal [27]. An example would be a man with a raised PSA (e.g. 4 ng/mL) who has a multi-parametric MRI that reveals no suspicious areas in a 120 cc prostate. In the context of the negative MRI carried out at an expert centre, knowledge that the PSA density is very low (0.03 ng/mL/cc) may influence the clinician to counsel the patient to avoid a prostate biopsy. Thus, mpMRI of the prostate can play a very important role in managing an elevated PSA in men with large prostates >100 cc.

4.1.1.1   PSA Kinetics in Large Prostates

In both BPH and prostate cancer, serial measurement of serum PSA can show increased readings over time, a phenomenon known as increased PSA velocity [28]. While PSA velocity tends to be higher in men with prostate cancer [28, 29], a trend towards a similar pattern may also be seen in men with benign prostates over 60 cc in volume [30]. Additionally, inflammation can lead to both dramatic PSA rises, and thus to very high PSA velocities [31], and to PSA fluctuation, whereby consecutive PSA readings oscillate between a range of values over time (for example, between 3 and 5). PSA fluctuation, possibly due to the connection between BPH and subclinical inflammation, is a feature frequently seen in men with BPH [28] and prostate volumes over 100 cc [32]. Therefore, PSA velocity may be a misleading marker in BPH, particularly in the very large prostate over 100 cc, and longitudinal assessment of PSA readings is essential to distinguish between increased PSA velocity and PSA fluctuation.

Many different formulas have been used to calculate PSA velocity [33, 34] and attempts have been made to simplify the concept by using alternative definitions, such as PSA doubling time (i.e. the time interval it takes for PSA to reach double its initial value) [28]. PSA sampling frequency and overall time period of observation have an effect on PSA velocity assessment [35], and a definitive cut off is yet to be defined. Similarly, controversy regarding the clinical value of using PSA kinetics has built up. While a systematic review concluded that PSA velocity is outperformed by elevated PSA as a trigger to decide whether a men should enter a prostate cancer diagnostic pathway [33], a more recent screening series with over 18,000 patients indicated that men have an increased risk of harbouring prostate cancer if they have two consecutive PSA velocity calculations above 0.4 ng/mL/year [29]. Despite the difference in opinions, experts seem to agree that longitudinal monitoring of PSA can aid clinical decision making and that, while PSA velocity should not be considered as a standalone marker, it can be a useful tool to tailor PSA surveillance in men without prostate cancer (i.e. men with higher PSA velocities should have a closer PSA follow up) [29, 34].

4.1.2 Free PSA in Large Prostates

PSA is produced as a proenzyme, proPSA. Thus, the molecule needs to be cleaved to become active. As PSA enters blood vessels, proteins bind to it in an effort to reduce its proteolytic activity (complexed PSA). ProPSA and inactive forms of PSA can circulate unbound (free PSA) [36]. Both complexed and free PSA can be accounted for when measuring total serum PSA but free PSA can also be read on its own. A low ratio between free and total PSA (free/total PSA) has been associated with prostate cancer due to mechanisms still to be thoroughly explained. A free/total ratio of less than 0.12 was initially defined as being associated with a higher risk of cancer [37, 38] but subsequent studies have proposed cut-offs of less than 0.25 [39–41]. At present, free/total PSA should only be used as a complement to total PSA [42], as different cut offs for the first may be needed in view of the magnitude of the second [43]. Similarly, free PSA fluctuates over time [42], so repeat readings may be necessary for accurate assessment of the ratio. Finally, free PSA may be increased in the presence of prostatic inflammation [3] (a phenomenon not uncommonly associated with BPH) and, in men with prostates over 40 cc in volume, free/total PSA may not help differentiate between BPH alone and prostate cancer [38], limiting the utility of this tool in men with large prostates and elevated PSA.

4.1.3 Prostate Cancer Screening Risk Stratification Tools That Incorporate Prostate Volume

A multitude of risk stratification tools have been developed with the aim of improving prostate cancer screening. A recent meta-analysis reviewed the most commonly studied and validated models [44]. Age, PSA and digital rectal examination (DRE) findings were factored into almost all tools and prostate volume (assessed using TRUS) was also taken into consideration in three of them: Prostata Class, the Finne model, and the European Randomized Study of Screening for Prostate Cancer (ERSPC) risk calculator (RC) 3 [44]. In ProstataClass [45], the Finne model [46], and the ERSPC RC 3 [47, 48], a higher prostate volume contributes to a lower likelihood of having prostate cancer. Conducting prostate volume assessments with TRUS may be burdensome, especially in primary care, but an additional analysis on the ERSPC model showed that estimating volume using DRE still increased predictive accuracy when compared to using only a combination of the other variables [48].

In this meta-analysis, ProstataClass and ERSPC RC 3 were the best performing models and their use showed improved accuracy in predicting the presence of cancer compared to using PSA values, DRE or prostate volume alone [44]. Despite this fact, screening risk stratification tools are still not systematically used in clinical practice and elevated serum PSA remains the main indication for prostate biopsy [49]. Given that these risk stratification tools were developed using cohorts with a median prostate volume between 30 and 50 cc [45, 46, 48], further analysis is needed to assess if there is benefit of using them in men with large prostates (over 100 cc in volume). Other PSA derivatives that have shown promise and may be useful adjuncts in guiding management decisions for biopsy in the large prostate include the prostate health index (PHI), which is a formula that combines total PSA, free PSA and [-2] proPSA, which has shown good performance in identifying high grade prostate cancer [50]. Additionally, Prostate Cancer Antigen 3 (PCA3), a urine based biomarker, may be particularly useful for guiding prostate biopsy decisions in the large prostate, as unlike PSA, its value is not thought to be associated with prostate volume [51].

4.1.4 Summary

Evidence is either insufficient or contradictory regarding the benefit of using PSA density, PSA transition zone density, PSA kinetics, free PSA, and risk stratification tools to help differentiate between BPH and cancer-bearing prostates in men with elevated serum PSA. To complicate things further, very limited data is available specifically for men with large prostates (over 100 cc). Today, clinical decision cannot be based solely on these factors, but in men with large prostates and elevated PSA levels the following seem to point to a lower likelihood of harbouring prostate cancer: presence of acute or chronic inflammation in previous biopsy [10, 52], low PSA density, low PSA transition zone density, null or low PSA velocity, long PSA doubling time, and high free/total PSA. Prostate mpMRI is one of the most promising modalities for men with a large prostate greater than 100 cc. Its use in conjunction with PSA may lead to improved discrimination of men that are likely to have prostate cancer and should proceed to prostate biopsy.

4.2 Biopsy Strategies in Men with Large Prostates

Men with large prostates are more likely to have increased serum PSA readings and thus, according to current guidelines, more prone to be offered a prostate biopsy to exclude prostate cancer [53]. This is particularly the case with prostates over the

100 cc volume threshold. Likewise, men with large prostates are more likely to have repeat prostate biopsies after a first negative result [54]. Evidence for the optimal biopsy strategy in men with big prostates is limited as they are often excluded from diagnostic trials.

Traditionally, prostate biopsies involved sextant transrectal prostate sampling under TRUS guidance. Since 1995, multiple publications reported that this biopsy scheme lead to prostate undersampling and consequently underdiagnosis of prostate cancer in large prostates (from 40 to over 80 cc in volume) [55–58]. Despite some authors advocating that sampling density had no effect on diagnosis [53], in 2006 it was established that 10–12 core TRUS guided biopsies should be advised due to higher malignancy detection rates compared to sextant biopsies [49, 59].

In large prostates, the matter of sampling density is even more controversial. Some studies imply that 10–12 transrectal biopsy cores may not be enough for large prostates [60] and that more intensive biopsy protocols should be used as first or second-line prostate biopsy options—either using saturation techniques [61] or biopsy schemes adjusted to prostate volume [62, 63]. Nevertheless, opposing evidence supports the concept that increasing the number of biopsy cores in large prostates may only contribute to higher diagnosis of clinically insignificant low volume Gleason 6 [54, 64] while carrying a higher adverse event rate [65]. Biopsy of large volume prostates is associated with more frequent haematuria, haematospermia, urinary retention, and pain [65], and these risks could potentially increase with more sampling intensive procedures.

An alternative way of increasing sampling density of larger prostates is to carry out transperineal template prostate biopsies (TTPB) using a brachytherapy grid [66]. This approach allows for a more systematic sampling of the prostate, with improved access to anterior and midline areas. Notwithstanding, it is resource intensive, requiring general or spinal anaesthetic [66], and, due to the increasing sampling, it is more prone to causing unwanted side effects [65]. Additionally, this strategy does not negate the problem of overdiagnosing insignificant cancer, but may maximise the identification of clinically significant cancer [67], which can be of value when clinical doubt exists.

Using the transrectal approach, due to limitations in needle length, it is often difficult to sample the anterior zone of large prostates. While the transperineal route can aid in sampling this area, sometimes the large prostate over 100 cc extends so much anteriorly that the biopsy needle hits the pubis as it is advanced through the biopsy template brachytherapy grid and through the perineum. The surgeon can perform certain maneuvers to help overcome this difficulty, such as flexing the hips by pushing the stirrups cranially, which helps raise the pubis giving more access for the biopsy needle to enter. In addition, the biopsy needle can be inserted freehand at an angle into the perineum by removing the brachytherapy grid, facilitating access to the anterior prostate.

Another way of balancing out adequate diagnosis and adverse events in larger prostates would be to use mpMRI-targeted biopsies. In these biopsies, the information obtained using mpMRI is used to influence conduct and placement of the needles. Recent evidence supports the use of mpMRI prior to biopsy [68] and this is becoming increasingly common practice as a means to identify suspicious areas that can then be biopsied. In the very large prostate a strategy of sampling only suspicious areas could be particularly advantageous. Even when using the trans-rectal route, pre-biopsy knowledge of the existence of a possible anterior tumour can aid in the sampling of the anterior prostate [69].

Overall, mpMRI-targeted biopsies appear to have better detection rates of clinically significant cancer than 12 core TRUS biopsy, with reduced diagnosis of clinically insignificant cancer [70]. Similarly, a prospective study in men who had targeted biopsy cores in addition to 12 core TRUS biopsies indicated that prostate cancer may be more likely to be diagnosed using targeted cores than systematic 12 core sampling in prostates with a volume from 40 up to 160 cc [71]. Compared to TTPB, mpMRI-targeted biopsies may have similar clinically significant cancer detection rates and lower clinically insignificant cancer detection rates [66]. They are also associated with fewer side effects [65].

Whilst early results would support the value of mpMRI-targeted biopsies over systematic biopsies in large prostates greater than 100 cc, further research is needed to elucidate its exact role. Variations in targeted biopsy practice exist, for example the method of registration used to carry out the biopsies can vary. A clear difference in detection rates between cognitive and software fusion targeted biopsies hasn't been found [72]. In experienced hands, cognitive targeted biopsy has shown good detection rates of cancer [66] whilst saving the expense of a software fusion system. However, the big prostate can be particularly challenging to perform targeted biopsy in and it is not known whether software assisted fusion may offer particular advantages over cognitive targeted biopsy in this group of men.

4.3   Conclusions

Currently, the prostate cancer diagnostic pathway still puts more value on total PSA than on multifactorial individual risk stratification. Research on PSA derived markers and risk stratification tools has failed to translate into clinical practice. As a result, many men with large prostates and elevated serum PSA but without prostate cancer are still being offered first and repeat prostate biopsies. This is a particular problem in men with very large prostates (greater than 100 cc), who are likely to have higher PSA levels independent of whether or not they harbor clinically significant prostate cancer.

A more conservative approach that is sensitive enough not to miss clinically significant cancer is needed. The use of mpMRI alone or in combination with previously studied markers may impart that change and serve as a useful tool in the assessment of the very large prostate. mpMRI has the potential to screen out men, leading to fewer prostate biopsies, and to guide a more accurate and less intense sampling by means of targeted biopsies. This may decrease the healthcare burden of suspected prostate cancer diagnostic pathways not only in terms of direct biopsy costs but also in terms of indirect costs that result from reducing both biopsy complications and intensive surveillance regimes due to fear of misdiagnosis.

References

1. Lilja H, Ulmert D, Vickers AJ. Prostate-specific antigen and prostate cancer: prediction, detection and monitoring. Nat Rev Cancer. 2008;8(4):268–78.
2. Roehrborn CG, Boyle P, Gould AL, Waldstreicher J. Serum prostate-specific antigen as a predictor of prostate volume in men with benign prostatic hyperplasia. Urology. 1999;53(3):581–9.
3. Gui-Zhong L, Libo M, Guanglin H, Jianwei W. The correlation of extent and grade of inflammation with serum PSA levels in patients with IV prostatitis. Int Urol Nephrol. 2011;43(2):295–301.
4. Berry SJ, Coffey DS, Walsh PC, Ewing LL. The development of human benign prostatic hyperplasia with age. J Urol. 1984;132(3):474–9.
5. Loeb S, Kettermann A, Carter HB, Ferrucci L, Metter EJ, Walsh PC. Prostate volume changes over time: results from the Baltimore Longitudinal Study of Aging. J Urol. 2009;182(4):1458–62.
6. Bianchi-Frias D, Vakar-Lopez F, Coleman IM, Plymate SR, Reed MJ, Nelson PS. The effects of aging on the molecular and cellular composition of the prostate microenvironment. PLoS One. 2010;5(9).
7. Roehrborn CG, McConnell J, Bonilla J, Rosenblatt S, Hudson PB, Malek GH, et al. Serum prostate specific antigen is a strong predictor of future prostate growth in men with benign prostatic hyperplasia. PROSCAR long-term efficacy and safety study. J Urol. 2000;163(1):13–20.
8. Pinsky PF, Kramer BS, Crawford ED, Grubb RL, Urban DA, Andriole GL, et al. Prostate volume and prostate-specific antigen levels in men enrolled in a large screening trial. Urology. 2006;68(2):352–6.
9. Park DS, Hong JY, Hong YK, Lee SR, Hwang JH, Kang MH, et al. Correlation between serum prostate specific antigen level and prostate volume in a community-based cohort: large-scale screening of 35,223 Korean men. Urology. 2013;82(6):1394–9.
10. Moreira DM, Nickel JC, Andriole GL, Castro-Santamaria R, Freedland SJ. Greater extent of prostate inflammation in negative biopsies is associated with lower risk of prostate cancer on repeat biopsy: results from the REDUCE study. Prostate Cancer Prostatic Dis. 2016;19(2):180–4.
11. Orsted DD, Bojesen SE, Nielsen SF, Nordestgaard BG. Association of clinical benign prostate hyperplasia with prostate cancer incidence and mortality revisited: a nationwide cohort study of 3,009,258 men. Eur Urol. 2011;60(4):691–8.
12. Stamey TA, Yang N, Hay AR, McNeal JE, Freiha FS, Redwine E. Prostate-specific antigen as a serum marker for adenocarcinoma of the prostate. N Engl J Med. 1987;317(15):909–16.
13. Benson MC, Whang IS, Olsson CA, McMahon DJ, Cooner WH. The use of prostate specific antigen density to enhance the predictive value of intermediate levels of serum prostate specific antigen. J Urol. 1992;147(3 Pt 2):817–21.
14. Benson MC, McMahon DJ, Cooner WH, Olsson CA. An algorithm for prostate cancer detection in a patient population using prostate-specific antigen and prostate-specific antigen density. World J Urol. 1993;11(4):206–13.
15. Meshref AW, Bazinet M, Trudel C, Aronson S, Peloquin F, Nachabe M, et al. Role of prostate-specific antigen density after applying age-specific prostate-specific antigen reference ranges. Urology. 1995;45(6):972–9.
16. Catalona WJ, Richie JP. deKernion JB, Ahmann FR, Ratliff TL, Dalkin BL, et al. Comparison of prostate specific antigen concentration versus prostate specific antigen density in the early detection of prostate cancer: receiver operating characteristic curves. J Urol. 1994;152(6 Pt 1):2031–6.
17. Al-Khalil S, Boothe D, Durdin T, Sunkara S, Watkins P, Yang S, et al. Interactions between benign prostatic hyperplasia (BPH) and prostate cancer in large prostates: a retrospective data review. Int Urol Nephrol. 2016;48(1):91–7.

18. Bare R, Hart L, McCullough DL. Correlation of prostate-specific antigen and prostate-specific antigen density with outcome of prostate biopsy. Urology. 1994;43(2):191–6.
19. Tanaka N, Fujimoto K, Chihara Y, Torimoto M, Hirao Y, Konishi N, et al. Prostatic volume and volume-adjusted prostate-specific antigen as predictive parameters for prostate cancer patients with intermediate PSA levels. Prostate Cancer Prostatic Dis. 2007;10(3):274–8.
20. Kang SH, Bae JH, Park HS, Yoon DK, Moon DG, Kim JJ, et al. Prostate-specific antigen adjusted for the transition zone volume as a second screening test: a prospective study of 248 cases. Int J Urol. 2006;13(7):910–4.
21. Kobayashi T, Kawahara T, Nishizawa K, Ogura K, Mitsumori K, Ide Y. Value of prostate volume measurement using transabdominal ultrasonography for the improvement of prostate-specific antigen-based cancer detection. Int J Urol. 2005;12(10):881–5.
22. Kurita Y, Ushiyama T, Suzuki K, Fujita K, Kawabe K. PSA value adjusted for the transition zone volume in the diagnosis of prostate cancer. Int J Urol. 1996;3(5):367–72.
23. Gregorio EP, Grando JP, Saqueti EE, Almeida SH, Moreira HA, Rodrigues MA. Comparison between PSA density, free PSA percentage and PSA density in the transition zone in the detection of prostate cancer in patients with serum PSA between 4 and 10 ng/mL. Int Braz J Urol. 2007;33(2):151–60.
24. Djavan B, Remzi M, Zlotta AR, Ravery V, Hammerer P, Reissigl A, et al. Complexed prostate-specific antigen, complexed prostate-specific antigen density of total and transition zone, complexed/total prostate-specific antigen ratio, free-to-total prostate-specific antigen ratio, density of total and transition zone prostate-specific antigen: results of the prospective multicenter European trial. Urology. 2002;60(4 Suppl 1):4–9.
25. Elliott CS, Shinghal R, Presti JC, Jr. The performance of prostate specific antigen, prostate specific antigen density and transition zone density in the era of extended biopsy schemes. J Urol 2008;179(5):1756-1761; discussion 61.
26. Peng Y, Shen D, Liao S, Turkbey B, Rais-Bahrami S, Wood B, et al. MRI-based prostate volume-adjusted prostate-specific antigen in the diagnosis of prostate cancer. J Magn Reson Imaging. 2015;42(6):1733–9.
27. Washino S, Okochi T, Saito K, Konishi T, Hirai M, Kobayashi Y, et al. Combination of PI-RADS score and PSA density predicts biopsy outcome in biopsy naive patients. BJU Int 2016;119(2):225–33.
28. Carter HB, Morrell CH, Pearson JD, Brant LJ, Plato CC, Metter EJ, et al. Estimation of prostatic growth using serial prostate-specific antigen measurements in men with and without prostate disease. Cancer Res. 1992;52(12):3323–8.
29. Loeb S, Metter EJ, Kan D, Roehl KA, Catalona WJ. Prostate-specific antigen velocity (PSAV) risk count improves the specificity of screening for clinically significant prostate cancer. BJU Int 2012;109(4):508-513; discussion 13–4.
30. Berger AP, Deibl M, Strasak A, Bektic J, Pelzer AE, Klocker H, et al. Large-scale study of clinical impact of PSA velocity: long-term PSA kinetics as method of differentiating men with from those without prostate cancer. Urology. 2007;69(1):134–8.
31. Eggener SE, Yossepowitch O, Roehl KA, Loeb S, Yu X, Catalona WJ. Relationship of prostate-specific antigen velocity to histologic findings in a prostate cancer screening program. Urology. 2008;71(6):1016–9.
32. Hobbs CP, Henderson JM, Malone PR. Living with a 100 ml prostate: Outcomes over a decade. J Clin Urol. 2014;8(3):202–8.
33. Vickers AJ, Savage C, O'Brien MF, Lilja H. Systematic review of pretreatment prostate-specific antigen velocity and doubling time as predictors for prostate cancer. J Clin Oncol. 2009;27(3):398–403.
34. Vickers AJ, Thompson IM, Klein E, Carroll PR, Scardino PT. A commentary on PSA velocity and doubling time for clinical decisions in prostate cancer. Urology. 2014;83(3):592–6.
35. Carter HB, Pearson JD, Waclawiw Z, Metter EJ, Chan DW, Guess HA, et al. Prostate-specific antigen variability in men without prostate cancer: effect of sampling interval on prostate-specific antigen velocity. Urology. 1995;45(4):591–6.

36. Mikolajczyk SD, Marks LS, Partin AW, Rittenhouse HG. Free prostate-specific antigen in serum is becoming more complex. Urology. 2002;59(6):797–802.
37. Pearson JD, Luderer AA, Metter EJ, Partin AW, Chan DW, Fozard JL, et al. Longitudinal analysis of serial measurements of free and total PSA among men with and without prostatic cancer. Urology. 1996;48(6A Suppl):4–9.
38. Moon DG, Yu JW, Lee JG, Kim JJ, Koh SK, Cheon J. The influence of prostate volume on the prostate-specific antigen (PSA) level adjusted for the transition zone volume and free-to-total PSA ratio: a prospective study. BJU Int. 2000;86(6):670–4.
39. Chun FK, Hutterer GC, Perrotte P, Gallina A, Valiquette L, Benard F, et al. Distribution of prostate specific antigen (PSA) and percentage free PSA in a contemporary screening cohort with no evidence of prostate cancer. BJU Int. 2007;100(1):37–41.
40. Capitanio U, Perrotte P, Zini L, Suardi N, Antebi E, Cloutier V, et al. Population-based analysis of normal Total PSA and percentage of free/Total PSA values: results from screening cohort. Urology. 2009;73(6):1323–7.
41. Pepe P, Aragona F. Incidence of insignificant prostate cancer using free/total PSA: results of a case-finding protocol on 14,453 patients. Prostate Cancer Prostatic Dis. 2010;13(4):316–9.
42. Ankerst DP, Gelfond J, Goros M, Herrera J, Strobl A, Thompson IM Jr, et al. Serial percent free prostate specific antigen in combination with prostate specific antigen for population based early detection of prostate cancer. J Urol. 2016;196(2):355–60.
43. Kitagawa Y, Ueno S, Izumi K, Kadono Y, Konaka H, Mizokami A, et al. Cumulative probability of prostate cancer detection in biopsy according to free/total PSA ratio in men with total PSA levels of 2.1-10.0 ng/ml at population screening. J Cancer Res Clin Oncol. 2014;140(1):53–9.
44. Louie KS, Seigneurin A, Cathcart P, Sasieni P. Do prostate cancer risk models improve the predictive accuracy of PSA screening? A meta-analysis. Ann Oncol. 2015;26(5):848–64.
45. Stephan C, Cammann H, Semjonow A, Diamandis EP, Wymenga LFA, Lein M, et al. Multicenter evaluation of an artificial neural network to increase the prostate cancer detection rate and reduce unnecessary biopsies. Clin Chem 2002;48(8):1279-1287.
46. Finne P, Finne R, Bangma C, Hugosson J, Hakama M, Auvinen A, et al. Algorithms based on prostate-specific antigen (PSA), free PSA, digital rectal examination and prostate volume reduce false-postitive PSA results in prostate cancer screening. Int J Cancer. 2004;111(2):310–5.
47. Roobol MJ, Steyerberg EW, Kranse R, Wolters T, van den Bergh RC, Bangma CH, et al. A risk-based strategy improves prostate-specific antigen-driven detection of prostate cancer. Eur Urol. 2010;57(1):79–85.
48. Roobol MJ, van Vugt HA, Loeb S, Zhu X, Bul M, Bangma CH, et al. Prediction of prostate cancer risk: the role of prostate volume and digital rectal examination in the ERSPC risk calculators. Eur Urol. 2012;61(3):577–83.
49. Mottet N, Bellmunt J, Bolla M, Briers E, Cumberbatch MG, Santis MD, et al. EAU guidelines on prostate cancer. http://uroweb.org/guideline/prostate-cancer/. Accessed October 2016.
50. Lazzeri M, Haese A, Abrate A, de la Taille A, Redorta JP, McNicholas T, et al. Clinical performance of serum prostate-specific antigen isoform [-2]proPSA (p2PSA) and its derivatives, %p2PSA and the prostate health index (PHI), in men with a family history of prostate cancer: results from a multicentre European study, the PROMEtheuS project. BJU Int. 2013;112(3):313–21.
51. Deras IL, Aubin SMJ, Blase A, Day JR, Koo S, Partin AW, et al. PCA3: A Molecular Urine Assay for Predicting Prostate Biopsy Outcome. J Urol. 2008;179(4):1587–92. doi: 10.1016/j. juro.2007.11.038. Epub 2008 Mar 4.
52. Porcaro AB, Novella G, Mattevi D, Bizzotto L, Cacciamani G, Luyk ND, et al. Chronic inflammation in prostate biopsy cores is an independent factor that lowers the risk of prostate cancer detection and is inversely associated with the number of positive cores in patients elected to a first biopsy. Curr Urol. 2016;9(2):82–92.
53. Ung JO, San Francisco IF, Regan MM, DeWolf WC, Olumi AF. The relationship of prostate gland volume to extended needle biopsy on prostate cancer detection. J Urol. 2003;169(1):130–5.

54. Pietzak EJ, Resnick MJ, Mucksavage P, Van Arsdalen K, Wein AJ, Malkowicz SB, et al. Multiple repeat prostate biopsies and the detection of clinically insignificant cancer in men with large prostates. Urology. 2014;84(2):380–5.
55. Uzzo RG, Wei JT, Waldbaum RS, Perlmutter AP, Byrne JC, Vaughan ED Jr. The influence of prostate size on cancer detection. Urology. 1995;46(6):831–6.
56. Karakiewicz PI, Bazinet M, Aprikian AG, Trudel C, Aronson S, Nachabe M, et al. Outcome of sextant biopsy according to gland volume. Urology. 1997;49(1):55–9.
57. Djavan B, Zlotta AR, Ekane S, Remzi M, Kramer G, Roumeguere T, et al. Is one set of sextant biopsies enough to rule out prostate Cancer? Influence of transition and total prostate volumes on prostate cancer yield. Eur Urol. 2000;38(2):218–24.
58. Basillote JB, Armenakas NA, Hochberg DA, Fracchia JA. Influence of prostate volume in the detection of prostate cancer. Urology. 2003;61(1):167–71.
59. Eichler K, Hempel S, Wilby J, Myers L, Bachmann LM, Kleijnen J. Diagnostic value of systematic biopsy methods in the investigation of prostate cancer: a systematic review. J Urol. 2006;175(5):1605–12.
60. Leibovici D, Shilo Y, Raz O, Stav K, Sandbank J, Segal M, et al. Is the diagnostic yield of prostate needle biopsies affected by prostate volume? Urol Oncol. 2013;31(7):1003–5.
61. Li YH, Elshafei A, Li J, Gong M, Susan L, Fareed K, et al. Transrectal saturation technique may improve cancer detection as an initial prostate biopsy strategy in men with prostate-specific antigen <10 ng/ml. Eur Urol. 2014;65(6):1178–83.
62. Ito K, Ohi M, Yamamoto T, Miyamoto S, Kurokawa K, Fukabori Y, et al. The diagnostic accuracy of the age-adjusted and prostate volume-adjusted biopsy method in males with prostate specific antigen levels of 4.1-10.0 ng/mL. Cancer. 2002;95(10):2112–9.
63. Eldred-Evans D, Kasivisvanathan V, Khan F, Hemelrijck MV, Polson A, Acher P, et al. The use of transperineal sector biopsy as a first-line biopsy strategy: a multi-institutional analysis of clinical outcomes and complications. Urol J. 2016;13(5):2849–55.
64. Chen ME, Troncoso P, Johnston D, Tang K, Babaian RJ. Prostate cancer detection: relationship to prostate size. Urology. 1999;53(4):764–8.
65. Borghesi M, Ahmed H, Nam R, Schaeffer E, Schiavina R, Taneja S, et al. Complications after systematic, random, and image-guided prostate biopsy. Eur Urol. 2017;71:353–65.
66. Kasivisvanathan V, Dufour R, Moore CM, Ahmed HU, Abd-Alazeez M, Charman SC, et al. Transperineal magnetic resonance image targeted prostate biopsy versus transperineal template prostate biopsy in the detection of clinically significant prostate cancer. J Urol. 2013;189(3):860–6.
67. Li YH, Elshafei A, Li J, Hatem A, Zippe CD, Fareed K, et al. Potential benefit of transrectal saturation prostate biopsy as an initial biopsy strategy: decreased likelihood of finding significant cancer on future biopsy. Urology. 2014;83(4):714–8.
68. Ahmed HU, El-Shater Bosaily A, Brown LC, Gabe R, Kaplan R, Parmar MK, et al. Diagnostic accuracy of multi-parametric MRI and TRUS biopsy in prostate cancer (PROMIS): a paired validating confirmatory study. Lancet. 2017;389(10071):815–22.
69. Haffner J, Lemaitre L, Puech P, Haber GP, Leroy X, Jones JS, et al. Role of magnetic resonance imaging before initial biopsy: comparison of magnetic resonance imaging-targeted and systematic biopsy for significant prostate cancer detection. BJU Int. 2011;108(8 Pt 2):E171–8.
70. Schoots IG, Roobol MJ, Nieboer D, Bangma CH, Steyerberg EW, Hunink MG. Magnetic resonance imaging-targeted biopsy may enhance the diagnostic accuracy of significant prostate cancer detection compared to standard transrectal ultrasound-guided biopsy: a systematic review and meta-analysis. Eur Urol. 2015;68(3):438–50.
71. de Gorski A, Roupret M, Peyronnet B, Le Cossec C, Granger B, Comperat E, et al. Accuracy of magnetic resonance imaging/ultrasound fusion targeted biopsies to diagnose clinically significant prostate cancer in enlarged compared to smaller prostates. J Urol. 2015;194(3):669–73.
72. Wysock JS, Rosenkrantz AB, Huang WC, Stifelman MD, Lepor H, Deng FM, et al. A prospective, blinded comparison of magnetic resonance (MR) imaging-ultrasound fusion and visual estimation in the performance of MR-targeted prostate biopsy: the PROFUS trial. Eur Urol. 2014;66(2):343–51.

Chapter 5
Medical Treatment of the Large Prostate

Nicholas Faure Walker and Jonathan Rees

5.1 Introduction

Men with large prostates are at increased risk of developing both voiding and storage lower urinary tract symptoms (LUTS) as well as acute and chronic urinary retention [1]. The precise risk of men with prostates over 100 mL in volume developing these conditions are not known but the Veterans Affairs (VA) cohort showed men with prostates over 30 mL in volume were three times more likely to develop acute urinary retention (AUR) [2], inferring that much larger glands are likely to be at a even greater risk. The Olmsted county study showed that men with prostates over 50 mL in volume were 3.5 times more likely to report moderate to severe LUTS than men with smaller prostates [3]. The probability of experiencing moderate to severe LUTS was also shown to be strongly correlated with age and a maximum urinary flow rate (Qmax) of less than 10 mL/s. The existing prospective studies including the VA cohort and Olmsted county included men with mean prostate volumes ranging from 36 to 55 mL [1–6]. Some of the studies also excluded men with PSA > 10 ng/mL which will have inevitably excluded many men with very large prostates. However, the PLESS study did look at a sub-group of men with mean prostate volumes of 82 mL [5].

Medical treatment for men with very large prostates aims to improve lower urinary tract symptoms (LUTS), and to prevent clinical progression, either in the form of deterioration of LUTS, the development of AUR or the need for surgery. Medications used in pursuit of this goal include 5α-reductase inhibitors, α-blockers, anti-muscarinics, β3-agonists, and phosphodiesterase inhibitors.

N.F. Walker (✉)
Guys Hospital, Great Maze Pond, London SE1 9RT, UK
e-mail: nicholas.faure.walker@gmail.com

J. Rees
Tyntesfield Medical Group, Bristol, North Somerset BS48 1BZ, UK
e-mail: drjonrees@gmail.com

© Springer International Publishing AG 2018   53
V. Kasivisvanathan, B. Challacombe (eds.), *The Big Prostate*,
https://doi.org/10.1007/978-3-319-64704-3_5

5.2 5α-Reductase Inhibitors (Table 5.1)

Benign prostatic hyperplasia (BPH) is likely to arise via a complex interaction between hormonal activation, growth factors and ageing [7]. Dihydrotestosterone is the hormone responsible for virilisation of the structures of the urogenital sinus. It has greater affinity for the androgen receptor than testosterone and is about twice as potent as testosterone. It is produced via reduction of testosterone by the lipophilic enzyme, 5α-reductase, which has two isoenzymes [8]: Type one is the dominant isoenzyme within sebaceous glands and found in the liver and skin as well as within the prostate where it is less abundant. Type two is the dominant isoenzyme within the prostate. The prostates of men with 5α-reductase deficiency are small and composed purely of stromal tissue unlike in unaffected males where there is also abundant epithelial tissue even though there is a greater proportion of stromal tissue compared to glandular tissue in men with BPH. It would appear that dihydrotestosterone has its principle effects in the stromal tissue and that glandular or epithelial hyperplasia occurs via paracrine rather than autocrine activation.

Dutasteride and Finasteride are both 4-aza steroid competitive inhibitors of 5α-reductase. Dutasteride inhibits both type one and type two 5α-reductase isoenzymes whereas Finasteride only inhibits the type two isoenzyme [9]. Nevertheless, Finasteride manages to reduce serum dihydrotestosterone by 70% and prostate dihydrotestosterone levels by up to 90% [8].

Finasteride was the first hormonal agent for treatment of BPH to be used in a placebo controlled randomised trial [10]. The results published in the New England Journal of Medicine in 1992 showed Finasteride was effective at reducing prostate volume, as well as improving LUTS and maximum urinary flow rate (Qmax) when compared to placebo. The VA cohort later demonstrated that Finasteride reduced prostate volume measured on trans-rectal ultrasound by 17% at 6 months which was maintained thereafter [11]. The subsequent MTOPS trial showed that Finasteride reduced the volume of prostates over 40 mL in volume by 19% compared to those in the Doxazosin and placebo arms, where the prostate volume increased by 24% over the same time period [1]. A later subset analysis of men with prostate volumes over 50 mL within the VA cohort showed that Finasteride decreased AUA symptom score by 3.6 points (1.1 more points than placebo) after 12 months of treatment. The PLESS study, an RCT of Finasteride versus placebo, was the first to follow men up for more than 1 year and lasted 4 years [4]. Patients had a mean prostate volume of 55 mL. The AUA (now IPSS) symptom scores were assessed every 4 months up to 4 years. The symptom scores of both the placebo and the Finasteride group decreased in a similar fashion over the first eight months. However, after 8 months, the symptom scores of the Finasteride group continued to decrease right up to the end of the study but the scores of the placebo group gradually increased from 8 months. Hence it would appear that Finasteride is marginally effective at improving LUTS in men with prostates over 50 mL in volume but the benefit is probably only evident after 8 months of treatment when compared to placebo. Whether there is an additional advantage in men with even larger prostates is not known.

Table 5.1 A summary of key studies of 5α-reductase Inhibitors in men with benign prostatic hyperplasia

Trial	Number of patients and trial design	Main inclusion/exclusion criteria	Intervention(s), length of study	Relevant outcomes
Finasteride trial (Gormley et al. 1992) [10]	895, RCT	Inclusion – Qmax <15 mL/s – BPH on DRE – Voided volume > 150 mL Exclusion – PSA > 40 µg/L – PVR > 350 mL – Neuropathic bladder	Finasteride (1 mg and 5 mg) or placebo 1 year	Prostate volume decreased by 19%, 18% and 3% in the 5 mg and 1 mg and placebo groups at 12 months Finasteride 5 mg showed a significantly greater decrease in symptom scores than placebo at 12 months but there was no difference to placebo at 3 months
VA (Lepor et al. 1996) [2]	1229, RCT	Inclusion: – 45–80 years – AUA symptom score ≥8 – 4 mL/s ≤ Qmax ≤15 mL/s – PVR < 300 mL Exclusion – Previous α-blocker use – Hormonal therapy in previous 3 months – Previous radiotherapy or pelvic surgery	Terazosin, Finasteride, combination, or placebo 1 year	Finasteride led to PV reduction of 17% at 26 weeks which was maintained Finasteride only showed an advantage over placebo at reducing symptom scores in men with prostates over 50 mL volume
PLESS (McConnell et al. 1998) [4]	3040, RCT	Inclusion: – Qmax <15 mL/s – BPE on DRE – Not taking α-blockers – Voided volume > 150 mL Exclusion: – PSA > 10 ng/mL – Precious use of α-blockers, hormonal therapy or anti-muscarinics – History of prostate cancer	Finasteride or placebo	Mean prostate size decreased in year 1 with no reduction thereafter Finasteride improved flow rate by 1.7 mL/s (vs. 0.2 mL/s in placebo) Finasteride reduced risk of needing surgery by 50% (ARR 5%) and developing AUR by 57% (ARR 4%) AUR or BPH surgery reported in 22% in highest prostate volume tertile (58–150 mL) and 8.9% of lowest for those on placebo; 74% RRR in highest tertile vs. 50% RRR with Finasteride

(continued)

Table 5.1 (continued)

Trial	Number of patients and trial design	Main inclusion/exclusion criteria	Intervention(s), length of study	Relevant outcomes
MTOPS (McConnell et al. 2003) [1]	3047, RCT	Inclusion: – ≥50 years – 8 ≤ AUA symptom score ≤ 30 – 4 mL/s ≤ Qmax ≤15 mL/s – Voided volume > 125 mL Exclusion: – Previous medical or surgical treatment for BPH – PSA > 10 ng/mL	Finasteride, Doxasozin, Combination, or Placebo 4.5 years	Finasteride reduced the volume of prostates over 40 mL in volume by 19% compared to those in the Doxazosin and placebo arms, where the prostate volume increased by 24% in the same time period Combination more effective than monotherapy in preventing clinical progression (66% reduction vs. 34% vs. 39%). Symptoms scores improved in all arms but most in combination AUR 0.6 per 100py with placebo, reduced to 0.2 (Finasteride) and 0.1 (combination) Finasteride and combination therapy reduced risk of requiring BPH surgery by 64 and 67%. Doxazosin did not reduce need for invasive therapy. The risk reduction was greater for men with prostate volumes >40 mL
CombAT (Roehrborn et al. 2011) [6]	4844, RCT	Inclusion: – ≥50 years – IPSS ≥12 – PV ≥ 30 mL – 1.5 ≤ PSA ≤ 10 – Voided volume > 125 mL Exclusion: – Prostate cancer – Previous invasive procedures to treat BPH – AUR within previous 3 months	Tamsulosin, Dutasteride or combination (no placebo) 4 years	Combined therapy more effective than Tamsulosin monotherapy at reducing risk of AUR or BPH related surgery if PV > 42 mL (benefit similar if PV > 57.8 mL but not statistically more) Symptom deterioration worse if baseline IPSS <20 or IPSS HRQL <4 Combination has greater effect in men with BMI ≥ 26.8

| PREDICT (Kirby et al. 2003) [25] | 3047, RCT | Inclusion:
– 50–80 years
– IPSS ≥12
– 5 mL/s ≤ Qmax ≤15 mL/s
– Voided volume > 150 mL
– BPH on DRE
Exclusion
– PSA > 10 ng/mL
– Previous invasive procedures for BPH
– PVR > 200 mL
– >1 episode of AUR in last year | Doxazosin, Finasteride, combination, or placebo
1 year | Doxazosin more effective than placebo and Finasteride at improving symptoms and Qmax. Combination therapy no more efficacious than Doxazosin monotherapy. No patients on combination therapy developed AUR or needed TURP compared to 7 in placebo group, 5 in Finasteride group and 1 in Doxazosin group |

The main role of a 5α-reductase inhibitors in men with large prostates is preventing AUR and the need for BPH surgery. The PLESS was the first study to assess AUR and BPH surgery as study endpoints [4, 5]. The patients in the PLESS study had large prostates with a mean volume of 55 mL. A later sub-set analysis by prostate size showed that 22% of men within the highest tertile, with a mean volume of 82 mL and a range between 58 and 150 mL, developed AUR or required BPH surgery compared to 8.9% in the lowest prostate volume tertile. Overall, 7% of men on placebo developed AUR compared to 4% of those on Finasteride; 10% of those on placebo required surgery compared to 5% of those on Finasteride. The greatest risk reduction in BPH surgery or AUR was seen in the highest prostate volume group. It therefore seems that men with the largest prostates have the most to benefit by early commencement of medical treatment with a 5AR.

The MTOPS study randomly assigned men with lower urinary tract symptoms to placebo, Doxazosin, Finasteride or combination therapy. Their primary endpoint was overall 'clinical progression' defined as an increase in four our more AUA symptom score points, acute urinary retention, urinary incontinence, renal insufficiency or recurrent urinary tract infection [1]. This was assessed at the time it was first observed within the 4.5 year follow up. Their secondary endpoints included invasive therapy for BPH. Finasteride was less effective than Doxazosin at reducing symptoms but more effective than placebo. Combination therapy was the most effective at reducing symptoms, preventing urinary retention and preventing surgery. Finasteride reduced the cumulative rate of urinary retention by 68% compared to placebo. The number needed to treat (NNT) to prevent one BPH surgery was 29 for Finasteride and 26 for combination therapy. However, the NNT was reduced to 23.1 and 15.9 by combination therapy for the subsets of men with PSA > 4.0 ng/mL and prostate volumes over 40 mL respectively. A post hoc analysis later showed that men with prostate volumes over 25 mL benefitted from Finasteride in terms of reducing clinical progression, urinary retention and the need for surgery [12].

The Combination of Avodart and Tamsulosin (CombAT) trial was the first to use Dutasteride (Avodart) rather than Finasteride. They excluded men with prostates less than 30 mL in volume hence their mean prostate volume of 55.0 mL was larger than most of the other studies except PLESS. There was no placebo arm. The incidence of AUR and BPH surgery was lower for all men treated with Dutasteride or combination compared to Tamsulosin independent of prostate volume, PSA, age, IPSS, Qmax, body mass index (BMI) and race. When the men were divided into tertiles, combination therapy was better than Tamsulosin monotherapy for reducing AUR and the need for BPH surgery in those with prostates between 42.0 and 57.8 mL and those with prostates over 57.8 mL. Although numerically superior, combined therapy was not statistically superior to Dutasteride monotherapy.

Men started on Finasteride and Dutasteride may be warned about erectile dysfunction, decreased libido and gynaecomastia. During the PREDICT trial, 5.8% of men on Finasteride and 3.3% of men on placebo reported erectile dysfunction. A large cohort with nested case control study in 2016 did not show significant erectile dysfunction attributable to 5α-reductase inhibitors [13]. Gynaecomastastia would appear to have an annual incidence of 0.1–0.5% [4, 14].

Overall it is clear from these studies that both Finasteride and Dutasteride can prevent AUR and BPH surgery in prostates over 25–40 mL. It is not clear whether there are additional advantages to men with prostates over this size but it seems likely from some of the sub-analyses of these larger prostate cohorts. However, men with larger prostates are at significantly higher risk of developing AUR and requiring surgery and so a 5α-reductase inhibitor would be an important first line treatment. There is no prospective evidence to show that there is any superiority of Finasteride over Dutasteride and retrospective studies do not warrant recommendation for one of these 5α-reductase inhibitors over the other [15].

5α-Reductase inhibitors are also used as treatment for haematuria arising from the prostate and to reduce bleeding during subsequent prostate surgery [16, 17]. In BPH, the microvascular density has been shown to be increased which may be the reason why BPH puts a patient at risk of prostatic bleeding [18]. Finasteride and Dutasteride reduce the microvascular density with the prostate [17]. A prospective study showed that recurrence of haematuria in men treated with Finasteride was reduced by 49% and none of the 17 men treated with Finasteride required surgery for haematuria compared to 7 (26%) of controls [16]. A randomised trial of a four weeks of Dutasteride, Finasteride or placebo before TURP showed that both 5α-reductase inhibitors reduced blood loss and the need for blood transfusions compared to placebo but there was no significant differences between Finasteride and Dutasteride [17]. Although 5α-reductase inhibitors have been shown to be beneficial in preventing bleeding during TURP, they have anecdotally been reported as making the prostate firmer and more difficult to morcellate during during holmium laser enucleation of the prostate (HoLEP).

Men with very large prostates often have raised PSA and hence may be under PSA surveillance owing to concerns over prostate cancer. As 5α-reductase inhibitors reduce prostate size, they also reduce PSA levels. A rise in PSA for a man on a 5α-reductase inhibitor can hence be more clinically concerning than in a man not on a 5α-reductase inhibitor. The degree of PSA rise has been shown to be linked to the likelihood of developing higher grade prostate cancer [19]. For the sake of monitoring, it is recommended that a man on a 5α-reductase inhibitor should have his PSA value doubled for comparison although any rise should trigger some concerns [20].

5.3 α-Blockers (Table 5.2)

Smooth muscle fibres make up approximately half the stroma of the prostate gland including the capsule. In BPH, the stromal and glandular tissue make up approximately 80 and 20% of the hyperplastic gland [7]. Unlike in female bladders, male bladder fibres become circular in orientation towards the bladder neck. This ring of muscle (the pre-prostatic sphincter) prevents retrograde ejaculation, by alpha-adrenergic modulated increased tone during erection and ejaculation. Despite its location, it does not appear to have any role in continence but BPH can lead to

Table 5.2 A summary of key studies of α-blockers in men with benign prostatic hyperplasia

Trial	Number of patients and trial design	Main inclusion/exclusion criteria	Intervention(s), length of study	Relevant outcomes
Phenoxybenzamine trial (Caine et al. 1978) [21]	50, RCT	Inclusion – BPH Exclusion – Renal failure arising from BPH – Evidence of cerebro-vascular disease	Phenoxybenzamine or placebo 14 days	Phenoxybenzamine increased Qmax by 6.2 mL/s compared to 1.2 mL/s for placebo No change in PVR Ejaculation problems reported in 8%
Tamsulosin trial (Lepor et al. 1998) [11]	756, RCT	Inclusion – ≥45 years – AUA symptom scire ≥13 – 4 mL/s ≤ Qmax ≤15 mL/s – PVR < 300 mL Exclusion – Finasteride treatment – Anticholinergic treatment – Cardiovascular or cerebrovascular disease – Previous surgery to urinary tract – Cancer of urinary tract	Tamsuloisn 0.4 mg, 0.8 mg or placebo 12 weeks	Qmax shown to improve after 4 h of Tamsulosin 0.4 mg Tamsulosin 0.4 mg improved AUA score by 8.3 (placebo 5.5) and Qmax by 1.75 mL/s (placebo 0.52 mL/s) at 12 week follow up Orthostatic hypotension similar in placebo and treatment groups
VA (Lepor et al. 1996) [2]	1229, RCT	Inclusion: – 45–80 years – AUA symptom score ≥8 – 4 mL/s ≤ Qmax ≤15 mL/s – PVR < 300 mL Exclusion – Previous α-blocker use – Hormonal therapy in previous 3 months – Previous radiotherapy or pelvic surgery	Terazosin, Finasteride, combination, or placebo 1 year	Terazosin more effective than Finasteride at reducing symptom scores and improving Qmax Qmax improvement with Terazosin peaked at 4 weeks Terazosin's effects independent of prostate size

MTOPS (McConnell et al. 2003) [1]	3047, RCT	Inclusion: – ≥50 years – 8 ≤ AUA symptom score ≤ 30 – 4 mL/s ≤ Qmax ≤15 mL/s – Voided volume > 125 mL Exclusion: – Previous medical or surgical treatment for BPH – PSA > 10 ng/mL	Finasteride, Doxasozin, Combination, or Placebo 4.5 years	Combination more effective than monotherapy in preventing 'clinical progression' (66% reduction vs. 34% vs. 39%). Symptoms scores improved in all arms but most in combination Doxazosin increased time to develop AUR but did not reduce incidence within 4 year follow up period Doxazosin did not reduce requirement for invasive therapy at 4 year follow up
Alfuzosin vs. Tamsulosin study (Hellstrom et al. 2006) [28]	166, RCT	Inclusion – Male 18–26 y – 'Normal' sexual function = IIEF ≥26 Exclusion: – Abnormal WHO 2003 semen analysis parameters	Tamsulosin, Alfuzosin, or placebo 5 days	Tamsulosin was associated with a 2.4 mL reduction in ejaculate volume after 5 days of treatment compared to Alfuzosin and placebo 35.4% of those on Tamsulosin (but none on Alfuzosin or placebo) reported anejaculation There was no difference in the urinary sperm concentration between the groups
CombAT (Roehrborn et al. 2011) [6]	4844, RCT	Inclusion: – ≥50 years – IPSS ≥12 – PV ≥ 30 mL – 1.5 ≤ PSA ≤ 10 – Voided volume > 125 mL Exclusion: – Prostate cancer – Previous invasive procedures to treat BPH – AUR within previous 3 months	Tamsulosin, Dutasteride or combination (no placebo) 1 year	Tamsulosin as effective as combination at preventing clinical deterioration if prostate volume < 40 mL

(continued)

Table 5.2 (continued)

Trial	Number of patients and trial design	Main inclusion/exclusion criteria	Intervention(s), length of study	Relevant outcomes
PrEDICT (Kirby et al. 2003) [25]	3047, RCT	Inclusion: – 50–80 years – IPSS ≥12 – 5 mL/s ≤ Qmax ≤15 mL/s – Voided volume > 150 mL – BPH on DRE Exclusion – PSA > 10 ng/mL – Previous invasive procedures for BPH – PVR > 200 mL – >1 episode of AUR in last year	Doxazosin, Finasteride, combination, or placebo 1 year	Doxazosin more effective than placebo and Finasteride at improving symptoms and Qmax Combination therapy no more efficacious than Doxazosin monotherapy No patients on combination therapy developed AUR or needed TURP compared to 7 in placebo group, 5 in Finasteride group and 1 in Doxazosin group

bladder outflow obstruction and LUTS [22]. Approximately 90% of the smooth muscle receptors are the α-1 subtype which mediate the contraction of smooth muscle within the prostate [23].

Phenoxybenzamine was the first α-blocker to be shown to improve LUTS in an RCT in 1978 though the only outcome measured used were day time and night time frequency and Qmax, which all improved. Phenoxybenzamine is a non-selective α-blocker and significant adverse effects including fatigue, dizziness, nasal congestion, hypotension and ejaculatory problems were reported in this trial.

The first selective α-1 blocker to be subjected to a randomised, placebo controlled trial was Terazosin (two, five or 10 mg) published by Lepor and colleagues in 1992 [24]. The mean prostate volume was 36.9 mL but outcomes of subsets of men with larger prostates were not assessed. The greatest benefit was seen in the 10 mg group with a 22.4% reduction in symptom score and a 24.4% increase in Qmax. The VA cohort study was the first to compare an α-blocker (Terazosin 10 mg) with a 5α-reductase inhibitor (Finasteride) and combination [2]. Terazosin was more effective at reducing symptoms scores and improving Qmax than Finasteride monotherapy, which was no more effective than placebo. The improvement in Qmax peaked at four weeks after starting Terazosin and the benefits were independent of prostate volume.

The PrEDiCT trial showed that Doxazosin (another α-1 blocker) was more effective than placebo and Finasteride at improving LUTS and that combination therapy was no more effective than Doxazosin monotherapy [25]. No patients on combination therapy developed AUR or required TURP compared to 7 in the placebo group, 5 in the Finasteride group and 1 in the Doxazosin group at 1 year. In the MTOPS trial, fewer patients on Doxazosin required BPH surgery or developed AUR at the end of the first year, but by 4.5 years follow up, Doxazosin was not found to prevent AUR or BPH surgery when compared to placebo [1].

Tamsulosin was the first sub-selective α-1a blocker to be trialled [26]. Although more selective for α-1a than α-1b, it had similar selectivity for α-1a and α-1d receptors [26]. A randomised placebo-controlled clinical trial of Tamsulosin at 400 and 800 μg showed that the 400 μg dose was effective at improving symptom scores and Qmax [27]. The onset of symptomatic improvement compared to placebo was observed after one week and improvement in Qmax was observed after the very first dose. The highest discontinuation rate was in the 800 μg arm (13%). The most commonly reported adverse events were rhinitis (12% vs. 6% on placebo) and abnormal ejaculation (6% on 400 μg, 18% on 800 μg and 0% for placebo). Although all patients showed a small drop in blood pressure, only 1% showed clinically significant orthostatic hypotension. The equivalent rates for postural hypotension for Doxazosin in other studies would appear to be between 4.0 and 5.8% [1, 25].

Tamsulosin 400 μg once daily was the first α-blocker that was effective at improving LUTS that did not require titration, which may partly explain its popularity [26]. A double blinded randomised study in 16–36 year old healthy volunteers given Alfuzosin, the latest α-1 blocker to enter the market, Tamsulosin 800 μg once daily or placebo showed Tamsulosin was associated with a 2.4 mL reduction in ejaculate volume compared to Alfuzosin and placebo [28]. The study reported that 35.4% of those of Tamsulosin who completed the study suffered from anejaculation rather than retrograde ejaculation. There was no significant difference in post ejaculation urinary sperm concentration between the groups suggesting the reduction in ejaculate did not arise from retrograde ejaculation. It was suggested that Tamsulosin impairs ejaculation as, unlike other α-blockers, it also inhibits $5HT_{1A}$ and D_3 receptors and can cross the blood-brain barrier and inhibit the central control of ejaculation. A randomised, placebo controlled trial of 15 and 10 mg doses of Alfuzosin showed Alfuzosin improved IPSS scores and Qmax without compromising blood pressure or ejaculatory function [29]. There does not appear to be an advantage of a 15 mg dose and so like Tamsulosin 400 μg once daily, titration is not required. There is no evidence specifically looking at the effectiveness of α-blockers in prostates of over 100 mL in volume. However, it would appear α-blockers are effective at improving Qmax from the very first dose, with maximum effect at 4 weeks. They also improve LUTS after a week of therapy with maximum effect at approximately four weeks for all prostate sizes. Alfuzosin 10 mg once daily avoids the need for dose titration like Tamsulosin 400 μg, but does not adversely affect ejaculation as frequently as Tamsulosin.

Men with large median lobes which indent the bladder are less likely to benefit from an alpha blocker [30, 31]. Protrusion of the prostate into the bladder is more common in men with larger prostates and the 'ball-valve' effect that results may be part of the reason for a lack of response to medical therapy [31]. Hence, a flexible cystoscopy is useful in patients who fail to respond to medical therapy as they may require BPH surgery.

There is some debate as to when to cease α-blockers for symptom control when they are used in combination with 5α-reductase inhibitors. The SMART-1 trial showed that most men's symptoms do not deteriorate if the α-blocker is stopped at 6 months of combination therapy [32]. A minority of patients in this study with severe symptoms (IPSS > 20), may have benefitted from longer term therapy. A sensible approach would be to follow up a patient after α-blocker withdrawal and simply re-start if the patient becomes symptomatic.

Although α-blockers may only defer a first episode of AUR rather than prevent it, they can increase the likelihood of spontaneous voiding following catheterization for AUR [33]. Following AUR, men given Alfuzosin for three days were 14% more likely to pass their trial without catheter compared to those on placebo. After 3 months of therapy, they were 8% less likely to require surgery. While the prevention of surgery in this short-term study is only minimal, an α-blocker is clearly a useful adjunct in helping a man become catheter free after developing AUR. It may also be prudent to give those men with larger prostates who are undergoing any form of surgery requiring catheterisation, a period of peri-operative alpha blockers to prevent the risk of retention.

5.4   Anti-muscarinics

LUTS in men may arise from bladder pathology as well as BPH [34]. The EPIC study showed that men and women suffered equally from overactive bladder (OAB) symptoms and the overall prevalence in the over 18's was 11.8% and the prevalence increased significantly with age in men [35]. Men with LUTS often find the storage symptoms such as frequency and urgency more bothersome than the voiding LUTS such as hesitancy and poor flow. The OAB symptoms can arise from the reduction in functional capacity from chronic urinary retention as a result of bladder outflow obstruction (BOO). However, the likelihood of men developing non-neurogenic detrusor overactivity on urodynamic studies also correlates well with age and degree of BOO [36]. The reason for this relationship is likely multi-factorial but it would appear that BOO leads to an increase in detrusor wall thickness with associated hypertrophy of neurons and changes in the bladder's electrophysiology [36].

The human bladder is innervated via parasympathetic fibres from the S2–4 nerve roots, which use acetylcholine for neurotransmission. Anti-muscarinic competitive acetylcholine antagonist medications are currently first line medical treatment for OAB symptoms (urgency, with or without urge incontinence, usually with frequency and nocturia) [37]. They aim to inhibit involuntary detrusor contractions during the bladder's storage phase that are believed to be at least partly responsible for these unpleasant symptoms. There is also evidence from animal studies that anti-muscarinic mediations may have some of their effects via reducing activity in unmyelinated c and Aδ fibres [38]. The key concern in using anti-muscarinics in men with very large prostates is that inhibition of detrusor contraction during voiding could lead to acute urinary retention or an increase in post void residual volumes, with worsening symptoms or even renal failure in the most extreme cases. Retrospective analyses have suggested there is an eight fold increased risk of AUR in the first 4 weeks of anti-muscarininic therapy with a two fold risk thereafter [39]. However, in a randomised, placebo controlled trial of Tamsulosin, Tolterodine or combination in men over 40 with BPH and OAB, the post void volume increased from a mean baseline of 53 by 5.3 mL for Tolterodine, 6.42 mL for combination and decreased by 3.6 mL for placebo after 12 weeks [40]. The differences were not statistically significant. AUR was reported in 0.4% of men on combination, 0.5% on Tolterodine and 0% for those on Tamsulosin monotherapy or placebo. This was a relatively short-term study and men with post void residual volumes of over 200 mL were excluded.

Anti-muscarinics should be used to help men with storage LUTS and BPH should certainly not automatically preclude men from their use. However, there is not enough reliable prospective, long-term data in men with very large prostates to conclude they will not contribute to poor emptying or even AUR. It is probably safe to use anti-muscarinics in this group of patients but a follow up post void volume at

12 weeks would be prudent until better evidence becomes available. Vesomni is a single daily tablet which contains combined Tamsulosin 400 μg and Solifenacin 6 mg. It can be a very useful medication for men with BOO and OAB symptoms.

5.5 β3-Agonists (Table 5.3)

Activation of the β3-adrenoreceptor via the cyclic adenosine monophosphate pathway by the neurotransmitter, noradrenaline, leads to dose dependent relaxation of the bladder during the storage phase in animal studies [41, 42]. In rodent models, activation of the β3 adrenoreceptor increases the period between voids and bladder compliance and does not compromise voiding function. The effects of β3 agonists may also result from inhibition of the pressure sensitive Aδ fibres and release of nitric oxide within the bladder epithelium leading to detrusor relaxation [43, 44]. Mirabegron was the first of these drugs to come to market and is helpful for patients who cannot tolerate the significant side effect profile of anti-muscarinics, such as dry mouth or who have conditions such as closed angle glaucoma, a history of recurrent falls or memory impairment which preclude anti-muscarinic therapy. Although their desired action is in the storage phase, it is conceivable that a β3 agonist could cause AUR or worsen voiding symptoms in men with very large prostates. The initial proof of concept study, the BLOSSOM trial, demonstrated that Mirabegron reduced urinary frequency, incontinence episodes, nocturia and improved quality of life outcome measures [45]. Improvements in symptoms were evident after 2 weeks and there was no significant change in post void volumes at the end of the 12 week study. The 38 men who were randomised were unlikely to be representative of men with very large prostates as men with clinically significant bladder outflow obstruction and post void volumes over 200 mL were excluded. Pooled data from the subsequent SCORPIO, ARIES and CAPRICORN trials with similar patient demographics showed that urinary retention occurred in no patients on Mirabegron 25 mg and 100 mg, 0.1% of patients on Mirabegron 50 mg compared to 0.4% on placebo and 0.6% on Tolterodine [46]. The PVR of all groups was non-significantly less at the end of the 12 week study than at baseline aside from Tolterodine where the mean PVR increased by 0.1 mL. The Symphony trial demonstrated Mirabegron's improvement of mean voided volume, frequency and urgency when used in combination with Solifenacin compared to Mirabegron monotherapy [47]. After 12 weeks, Mirabegron increased the mean PVR by 0.2 mL when used as monotherapy and by 10.7 mL when used in combination. There was concern that a β-agonist mediation could cause a tachycardia but the mean heart rate increased by 1.0 beats per minute after 12 weeks.

β3 Agonists may be useful in conjunction with or as a substitute for anticholinergics. They do not appear to significantly impede voiding but it is not clear if this is the case for men with high post void residuals. Until more reliable data is available for men with bladder outflow obstruction and β3 agonists, a review of a patient at risk of developing retention with a follow up PVR measurement at 12 weeks would appear prudent.

Table 5.3 A summary of key studies of β3-agonists in men with benign prostatic hyperplasia

Trial	Number of patients and trial design	Main inclusion/exclusion criteria	Intervention(s), follow up	Relevant outcomes
BLOSSOM trial (Chapple et al. 2013) [45]	314, RCT	Inclusion – ≥18 (male and female) – OAB symptoms for >3 months – Average micturition frequency ≥ 8× per day, and ≥3 episodes of urgency within 3 days Exclusion – Clinically significant outflow obstruction – PVR > 200 mL – Predominant stress urinary incontinence – Neuropathic bladder – Self-catheterisation – Previous pelvic radiation – Contra-indications to anti-cholinergics	Mirabegron 100 or 150 mg, Tolterodine 4 mg, or placebo 4 weeks	Mirabegron 100 mg and 150 mg reduced urgency and incontinence episodes by 2.3 and 2.2 episodes per day (1.5 less for Tolterodine and 1.0 less for placebo) Mirabegron improved nocturia episodes by 0.6 per 24 h (0.2 for placebo) Symptoms improved after 2 weeks No change in PVR woth Mirabegron Mirabegron 150 mg caused a 5 bpm increase in heart rate
Pooled analysis of SCORPIO, ARIES and CAPRICORN trials (Nitti 2013) [46]	3542, polled analysis of 3 RCT's	Inclusion – ≥18 (male and female) – OAB symptoms for >3 months – Average micturition frequency ≥ 8× per day, and ≥3 episodes of urgency within 3 days Exclusion – Daily urine output >3 L – Predominant stress urinary incontinence	Mirabegron 25 mg, 50 mg or 100 mg, or placebo Tolterodine also included in one trial 12 weeks	Mirabegron 50 mg and 100 mg reduced mean incontinence episodes by 1.49 and 1.50 per day (placebo −1.1). Mean micturitions per day were reduced by 1.75 and 1.74 by Mirabegron 50 mg and 100 mg (placebo reduced daily micturitions by 1.2) Urinary retention seen in 0.5% patients on placebo, <0.1%on Mirabegron 50 mg and in no patients on Mirabegron 25 mg and 100 mg Increases of ≥150 mL PVR were seen in 0.7% of those on placebo, 0% on Mirabegron 25 mg, 0.3% Mirabegron 50 mg, 0.4% Mirabegron 100 mg and 0.8% on Tolterodine. All groups had a non-statistically significant fall from baseline PVR

(continued)

Table 5.3 (continued)

Trial	Number of patients and trial design	Main inclusion/exclusion criteria	Intervention(s), follow up	Relevant outcomes
Symphony trial (Abrams et al. 2015) [47]	1306, RCT	Inclusion – ≥18 (male and female) – OAB symptoms for >3 months	Solifenacin 2.5, 5, or 10 mg, Mirabegron 25, combinations, or placebo 12 weeks	Mean micturitions per day decreased significantly with with Solifenacin and all doses of Mirabegron All treatment groups (inc placebo) demonstrated a reduction in incontinence episodes from baseline to the end of the study. Only Solifenacin 5 mg with Mirabegron 25 mg showed an improvement compared to Solifencin 5 mg monotherapy None of the Mirabegron monotherapy groups developed acute urinary retention The largest gain in PVR over the study period was seen in the Solifenacin 10 mg with Mirabegron 50 mg group (13.9 mL) Heart rate increased in patients on Mirabegron 50 mg by 1.0 bpm at the end of the study

5.6   Phosphodiesterase Inhibitors

Phosphodiesterase 5 inhibitors (PDE5-I) are best known in urology for treating erectile dysfunction by increasing blood flow into the corpora cavernosa. Following neural stimulation, nitric oxide (NO) activates guanylate cyclase which converts GTP into cyclic guanosine monophosphate (cGMP) which in turn activates cGMP dependent kinase phosphorylating several proteins leading to trabecular and arterial smooth muscle relaxation [48]. This leads to arterial dilatation, venous constriction and improved turgidity of erections.

PDE5 is found in the arterial smooth muscle of the lungs and PDE5-I were first brought to market for treatment of hypertension and angina and are now used as treatment for pulmonary hypertension [49]. PDE5-I have been shown in several trials to improve LUTS (both storage and voiding) and to marginally improve Qmax. The aetiology of its beneficial effects on LUTS are complex and likely multi-factorial [50] but thought to be related to increased pelvic blood flow. Relaxation of the PDE5-dependent smooth muscle found within the bladder neck, detrusor muscle, prostate and urethra may be responsible for the improved voiding and storage symptoms reported in several trials [51, 52]. There is also abundant PDE5 within the inferior vesicular artery and its branches to the prostate and urethra [50]. It is possible that PDE5-I improve blood flow to these organs. LUTS have been linked to the metabolic syndrome and hypertension resulting in poor oxygenation of these organs leading to fibrosis, contractile changes and increases in urethral resistance. However, it would seem unlikely that all the improvements in LUTS are from counteraction of these chronic processes as the improvements in LUTS with PDE5-I are observed within one week [52]. Moreover it is likely that PDE5-I have an effect on the afferent pathways as well [50]. In rat models, cGMP and PDE5-I led to an increase in the intervals between bladder contractions and an increase in the micturition pressure threshold suggesting inhibition of the afferent pathways [53].

Only one RCT has compared a PDE5-I (Tadalafil 5 mg) with an α-blocker (Tamsulosin 400μg) and placebo [52]. This showed improvements for both Tamsulosin and Tadalafil compared to placebo in Qmax and voiding symptoms. There was numerical improvement in storage symptoms at 12 weeks (p = 0.055). There was no statistically significant difference between Tamsulosin and Tadalafil for these outcomes. The PVR for patients on placebo, Tadalafil and Tamsulosin fell by 1.2, 4.6 and 10.2 mL at the end of the study. These changes were not statistically significant but it is unlikely they would lead to acute or chronic urinary retention.

PDE5-I are now recommended and licensed for the treatment of male LUTS though there is no longer term data to confirm their safety or their ability to prevent progression [54]. Tadalafil 5 mg appears an effective treatment for male LUTS and would be particularly appropriate for men who also suffer from erectile dysfunction. There is a strong correlation between the severity of LUTS and erectile dysfunction in the ageing male and so men with very large prostates may well be seeking concomitant treatment for LUTS and ED [55]. Hopefully, future studies will compare its effectiveness and safety by means of a RCT against placebo, α-blockers, 5α-reductase inhibitors alone and in combination.

5.7 Indications for Surgery

When LUTS are still bothersome despite medical therapy and there are signs of bladder outflow obstruction, patients should be offered surgery depending on their co-morbidities. Similarly, patients who have had an episode of urinary retention and have not managed to void without a catheter should also be offered surgery. Particular attention should be given to those with significant median lobes and prostatic indentation of the bladder, as they are unlikely to respond to α-blockers and surgery would offer a better chance of symptomatic improvement and it is not known how effective 5α-reductase inhibitors are for this subset of patients [30].

Men may prefer a definitive surgical procedure rather than up to three daily medications to treat their symptoms or their concern that they may develop AUR. Depending on the likely length of medical treatment, surgical intervention may also offer long term cost savings.

Strong indications for BPH surgery rather than medical therapy in large prostates include chronic urinary retention with renal insufficiency (high pressure chronic urinary retention), the presence of bladder stones, recurrent acute urinary retention with evidence of bladder outflow obstruction and haematuria arising from the prostate refractory to 5α reductase inhibitor therapy [54]. Ultimately, medical therapies have an important role in the initial management of men with LUTS and a very enlarged prostate but this group of men will often require bladder outflow surgery if they progress.

5.8 Conclusion

Men with very large prostates are at a high risk of experiencing severe storage and voiding LUTS, developing acute and chronic urinary retention and requiring surgery. Symptoms are likely to be helped quickly by α-blockers such as Alfuzosin and Tamsulosin unless there is significant indentation of the bladder by a very large prostate. These α-blockers are probably as effective as a daily PDE5-I which would also help treat concomitant ED. 5α-reductase inhibitors will help improve symptoms after several months of treatment but their main role is to prevent acute urinary retention and the requirement for surgery which is particularly relevant to men with very large prostates.

References

1. McConnell JD, et al. The long-term effect of doxazosin, finasteride, and combination therapy on the clinical progression of benign prostatic hyperplasia. N Engl J Med. 2003;349:2387–98.
2. Lepor H, et al. The efficacy of terazosin, finasteride, or both in benign prostatic hyperplasia. Veterans Affairs Cooperative Studies Benign Prostatic Hyperplasia Study Group. N Engl J Med. 1996;335:533–9.

3. Girman CJ, et al. Natural history of prostatism: relationship among symptoms, prostate volume and peak urinary flow rate. J Urol. 1995;153:1510–5.
4. McConnell JD, et al. The effect of finasteride on the risk of acute urinary retention and the need for surgical treatment among men with benign prostatic hyperplasia. Finasteride Long-Term Efficacy and Safety Study Group. N Engl J Med. 1998;338:557–63.
5. Roehrborn CG, et al. Serum prostate-specific antigen concentration is a powerful predictor of acute urinary retention and need for surgery in men with clinical benign prostatic hyperplasia. PLESS Study Group. Urology. 1999;53:473–80.
6. Roehrborn CG, et al. Clinical outcomes after combined therapy with dutasteride plus tamsulosin or either monotherapy in men with benign prostatic hyperplasia (BPH) by baseline characteristics: 4-year results from the randomized, double-blind Combination of Avodart and Tamsulosin (CombAT) trial. BJU Int. 2011;107:946–54.
7. Bartsch G, Rittmaster RS, Klocker H. Dihydrotestosterone and the concept of 5alpha-reductase inhibition in human benign prostatic hyperplasia. World J Urol. 2002;19:413–25.
8. Bartsch G, Rittmaster RS, Klocker H. Dihydrotestosterone and the concept of 5alpha-reductase inhibition in human benign prostatic hyperplasia. Eur Urol. 2000;37:367–80.
9. Nickel JC. Comparison of clinical trials with finasteride and dutasteride. Rev Urol. 2004;6(Suppl 9):S31–9.
10. Gormley GJ, et al. The effect of finasteride in men with benign prostatic hyperplasia. The Finasteride Study Group. N Engl J Med. 1992;327:1185–91.
11. Lepor H, Williford WO, Barry MJ, Haakenson C, Jones K. The impact of medical therapy on bother due to symptoms, quality of life and global outcome, and factors predicting response. Veterans Affairs Cooperative Studies Benign Prostatic Hyperplasia Study Group. J Urol. 1998;160:1358–67.
12. Kaplan, S. A. et al. Combination therapy with doxazosin and finasteride for benign prostatic hyperplasia in patients with lower urinary tract symptoms and a baseline total prostate volume of 25 mL or greater. J. Urol. 2006;175, 217–20; discussion 220–1.
13. Hagberg KW, Divan HA, Persson R, Nickel JC, Jick SS. Risk of erectile dysfunction associated with use of 5-α reductase inhibitors for benign prostatic hyperplasia or alopecia: population based studies using the Clinical Practice Research Datalink. BMJ. 2016;354:i4823.
14. Haillot O, et al. The effects of combination therapy with dutasteride plus tamsulosin on clinical outcomes in men with symptomatic BPH: 4-year post hoc analysis of European men in the CombAT study. Prostate Cancer Prostatic Dis. 2011;14:302–6.
15. DerSarkissian M, et al. Comparing Clinical and Economic Outcomes Associated with Early Initiation of Combination Therapy of an Alpha Blocker and Dutasteride or Finasteride in Men with Benign Prostatic Hyperplasia in the United States. J Manag Care Spec Pharm. 2016;22:1204–14.
16. Foley SJ, et al. A prospective study of the natural history of hematuria associated with benign prostatic hyperplasia and the effect of finasteride. J Urol. 2000;163:496–8.
17. Bansal A, Arora A. Transurethral resection of prostate and bleeding: a prospective randomized, double blind, placebo controlled trial to see efficacy of short term use of finasteride and dutasteride on operative blood loss and prostatic micro-vessel density. J Endourol. 2017. doi: 10.1089/end.2016.0696-rev
18. Foley SJ, Bailey DM. Microvessel density in prostatic hyperplasia. BJU Int. 2000;85:70–3.
19. Marberger M, et al. Usefulness of prostate-specific antigen (PSA) rise as a marker of prostate cancer in men treated with dutasteride: lessons from the REDUCE study. BJU Int. 2012;109:1162–9.
20. Pannek J, et al. Influence of finasteride on free and total serum prostate specific antigen levels in men with benign prostatic hyperplasia. J Urol. 1998;159:449–53.
21. Caine M, Perlberg S, Meretyk S. A placebo-controlled double-blind study of the effect of phenoxybenzamine in benign prostatic obstruction. Br J Urol. 1978;50:551–54.
22. Mundy AR, Fitzpatrick J, Neal DE, George NJR. The scientific basis of urology. 2nd ed. Boca Raton: CRC; 2004.

23. Lepor H, Gup DI, Baumann M, Shapiro E. Laboratory assessment of terazosin and alpha-1 blockade in prostatic hyperplasia. Urology. 1988;32:21–6.
24. Lepor H, et al. A randomized, placebo-controlled multicenter study of the efficacy and safety of terazosin in the treatment of benign prostatic hyperplasia. J Urol. 1992;148:1467–74.
25. Kirby RS, et al. Efficacy and tolerability of doxazosin and finasteride, alone or in combination, in treatment of symptomatic benign prostatic hyperplasia: the Prospective European Doxazosin and Combination Therapy (PREDICT) trial. Urology. 2003;61:119–26.
26. Lepor H. Alpha blockers for the treatment of benign prostatic hyperplasia. Rev Urol. 2007;
27. Lepor H. Phase III Multicenter Placebo-Controlled Study of Tamsulosin in Benign Prostatic Hyperplasia. Urology. 1998;51:892–900.
28. Hellstrom WJG, Sikka SC. Effects of Acute Treatment With Tamsulosin Versus Alfuzosin on Ejaculatory Function in Normal Volunteers. J Urol. 2006;176:1529–33.
29. Roehrborn CG. Efficacy and safety of once-daily alfuzosin in the treatment of lower urinary tract symptoms and clinical benign prostatic hyperplasia: a randomized, placebo-controlled trial. Urology. 2001;58:953–9.
30. Lebdai, S. et al. [Clinical impact of the intravesical prostatic protrusion: a review by the LUTS Committee of the French Urological Association]. Prog Urol. 2014;24, 313–8.
31. Seo YM, Kim HJ. Impact of intravesical protrusion of the prostate in the treatment of lower urinary tract symptoms/benign prostatic hyperplasia of moderate size by alpha receptor antagonist. Int Neurourol J. 2012;16:187–90.
32. Barkin J, et al. Alpha-blocker therapy can be withdrawn in the majority of men following initial combination therapy with the dual 5alpha-reductase inhibitor dutasteride. Eur Urol. 2003;44:461–6.
33. McNeill SA, Hargreave TB, Roehrborn CG. Alfuzosin 10 mg once daily in the management of acute urinary retention: Results of a double-blind placebo-controlled study. Urology. 2005;65:83–9.
34. Chapple, C. Systematic review of therapy for men with overactive bladder. Can Urol Assoc J. 2011;5(5 Suppl 2): S143–5.
35. Irwin DE, et al. Population-based survey of urinary incontinence, overactive bladder, and other lower urinary tract symptoms in five countries: results of the EPIC study. Eur Urol. 2006;50:1306–15.
36. Oelke M, et al. Age and bladder outlet obstruction are independently associated with detrusor overactivity in patients with benign prostatic hyperplasia. Eur Urol. 2008;54:419–26.
37. Abrams, P., Cardozo, L., Fall, M., Griffiths, D. & Rosier, P.; Standardisation Subcommittee of the International Continence Society. The standardisation of terminology of lower urinary tract function: report from the Standardisation Sub-committee of the International Continence Society. Neurourol Urodyn. 2002;21(2):167–78.
38. De Laet K, De Wachter S, Wyndaele JJ. Systemic oxybutynin decreases afferent activity of the pelvic nerve of the rat: New insights into the working mechanism of antimuscarinics. Neurourol Urodyn. 2006;25:156–61.
39. Martín-Merino E, García-Rodríguez LA, Massó-González EL, Roehrborn CG. Do oral antimuscarinic drugs carry an increased risk of acute urinary retention? J Urol. 2009;182:1442–8.
40. Kaplan SA, et al. Tolterodine and Tamsulosin for Treatment of Men With Lower Urinary Tract Symptoms and Overactive Bladder: A Randomized Controlled Trial. JAMA. 2006;296:2319–28.
41. Sadananda P, Drake MJ, Paton JFR, Pickering AE. A functional analysis of the influence of $\beta3$-adrenoceptors on the rat micturition cycle. J Pharmacol Exp Ther. 2013;347:506–15.
42. Chapple CR, Cardozo L, Nitti VW, Siddiqui E, Michel MC. Mirabegron in overactive bladder: A review of efficacy, safety, and tolerability. NeurourolUrodyn. 2014;33:17–30.
43. Aizawa N, Igawa Y, Nishizawa O, Wyndaele JJ. Effects of CL316,243, a beta 3-adrenoceptor agonist, and intravesical prostaglandin E2 on the primary bladder afferent activity of the rat. NeurourolUrodyn. 2010;29:771–6.

44. Vij M, Drake MJ. Clinical use of the β3 adrenoceptor agonist mirabegron in patients with overactive bladder syndrome. Ther Adv Urol. 2015;7:241–8.
45. Chapple CR, et al. A proof-of-concept study: Mirabegron, a new therapy for overactive bladder. NeurourolUrodyn. 2013;32:1116–22.
46. Nitti VW, et al. Mirabegron for the treatment of overactive bladder: a prespecified pooled efficacy analysis and pooled safety analysis of three randomised, double-blind, placebo-controlled, phase III studies. Int J Clin Pract. 2013;67:619–32.
47. Abrams P, et al. Combination treatment with mirabegron and solifenacin in patients with overactive bladder: efficacy and safety results from a randomised, double-blind, dose-ranging, phase 2 study (Symphony). Eur Urol. 2015;67:577–88.
48. Corbin JD. Mechanisms of action of PDE5 inhibition in erectile dysfunction. Int J Impot Res. 2004;16(Suppl 1):S4–7.
49. Ghofrani HA, Osterloh IH, Grimminger F. Sildenafil: from angina to erectile dysfunction to pulmonary hypertension and beyond. Nat Rev Drug Discov. 2006;5:689–702.
50. Giuliano F, et al. The mechanism of action of phosphodiesterase type 5 inhibitors in the treatment of lower urinary tract symptoms related to benign prostatic hyperplasia. Eur Urol. 2013;63:506–16.
51. Egerdie RB, et al. Tadalafil 2.5 or 5 mg administered once daily for 12 weeks in men with both erectile dysfunction and signs and symptoms of benign prostatic hyperplasia: results of a randomized, placebo-controlled, double-blind study. J Sex Med. 2012;9:271–81.
52. Oelke M, et al. Monotherapy with tadalafil or tamsulosin similarly improved lower urinary tract symptoms suggestive of benign prostatic hyperplasia in an international, randomised, parallel, placebo-controlled clinical trial. Eur Urol. 2012;61:917–25.
53. Caremel R, Oger-Roussel S, Behr-Roussel D, Grise P, Giuliano FA. Nitric oxide/cyclic guanosine monophosphate signalling mediates an inhibitory action on sensory pathways of the micturition reflex in the rat. Eur Urol. 2010;58:616–25.
54. Gratzke C, et al. EAU guidelines on the assessment of non-neurogenic male lower urinary tract symptoms including benign prostatic obstruction. Eur Urol. 2015;67:1099–109.
55. Rosen R, et al. Lower urinary tract symptoms and male sexual dysfunction: the multinational survey of the aging male (MSAM-7). Eur Urol. 2003;44:637–49.

Chapter 6
Surgical Treatment: Prostate Artery Embolization

Tiago Bilhim, João Pisco, Lúcia Fernandes, Nuno Vasco Costa, and António Gouveia Oliveira

6.1 Rationale of PAE for BPH

The main goal when treating patients with benign prostatic hyperplasia (BPH) is to relieve lower urinary tract symptoms (LUTS) related to bladder outlet obstruction (BOO). LUTS are believed to be due to two main components: (1) Static due to urethral obstruction by an enlarged prostate (thus, many clinicians prefer to use the terms BPO—benign prostatic obstruction or BPE—benign prostatic enlargement) and (2) Dynamic due to increased prostatic smooth muscle tone. It is important, however, to note that LUTS are multifactorial, and may be due to non-prostatic diseases as bladder dysfunction, urethral strictures or cardiac disease. Thus, it is essential to rule out non-prostatic causes of LUTS, that even though less frequent, may mimic BPH-related LUTS.

Prostate artery embolization (PAE) leads to prostate tissue necrosis and intends to target the two components of BPH-related LUTS: (1) static—through the destruction of peri-urethral prostate tissue relieving the urethral obstruction with an overall reduction in prostate size; (2) dynamic—through the destruction of α1-adrenergic receptors in the prostatic stroma leading to decreased prostatic smooth muscle tone. Also, the PAE-induced local ischemia may lead to an immediate activation of nitric oxide (NO) synthase and subsequent overproduction of NO in the prostate, thus lowering smooth muscle tone and BOO-related LUTS [1].

T. Bilhim, M.D., Ph.D., E.B.I.R. (✉) • L. Fernandes, M.D. • N.V. Costa, M.D.
Nova Medical School, Lisbon, Portugal

Saint Louis Hospital, Lisbon, Portugal
e-mail: tiagobilhim@hotmail.com; luci_fernandes@hotmail.com; nunovpc@gmail.com

J. Pisco, M.D., Ph.D.
Saint Louis Hospital, Lisbon, Portugal
e-mail: martinspisco@hslouis.pt

A.G. Oliveira, M.D., Ph.D.
Departamento de Farmácia, Universidade Federal do Rio Grande do Norte, Natal, Brazil
e-mail: oliveira.amg@gmail.com

© Springer International Publishing AG 2018
V. Kasivisvanathan, B. Challacombe (eds.), *The Big Prostate*,
https://doi.org/10.1007/978-3-319-64704-3_6

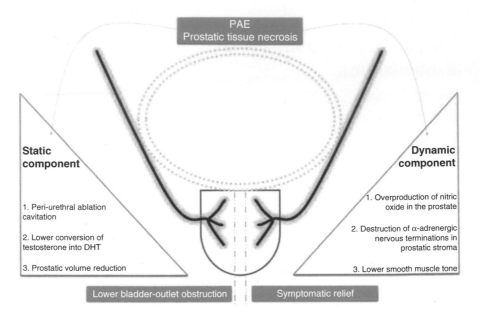

Fig. 6.1 Rationale of prostate artery embolization (PAE) for benign prostatic hyperplasia (BPH). *DHT* dihydrotestosterone

The prostate tissue is also responsible for the conversion of testosterone into dihydrotestosterone (DHT) and transportation of DHT into the gland. DHT is the chief hormone leading to prostate growth with age. Thus, with prostate tissue destruction the ability to convert testosterone into DHT becomes compromised leading to slower prostate tissue growth with time. Both components are believed to relieve BOO and related LUTS (Fig. 6.1).

The static component of LUTS has traditionally been treated with 5α-reductase inhibitors and/or surgery to reduce prostate volume, prostate-induced urethral obstruction and BOO-related LUTS. Six months after starting treatment with 5α-reductase inhibitors there is a mean prostate volume reduction of 20–30% with a mean prostate-specific-antigen (PSA) reduction of 40–50% [2]. These figures are similar to those obtained 6 months after PAE, reinforcing the potential role of PAE as an effective tool to block the functional androgen-signalling axis [1]. The dynamic component of BPH-related LUTS has traditionally been treated with α-blockers that improve LUTS 30–40% with an increase in peak urinary flow rate (Qmax) of 15–30% [2]. More recently, the dynamic component of BPH-related LUTS has also been treated with phosphodiesterase type 5 inhibitors (PDE5-Is) that lead to lower smooth muscle tone inside the prostate through the activation of the NO-pathway. Treatment with PDE5-Is has shown to lead to LUTS relief of six points, with no significant effect on Qmax [2]. These figures are somewhat inferior to PAE, probably because PAE leads to LUTS-BOO relief through both static and dynamic components involving all these potential pathways.

6.2 Technical Steps

PAE planning starts with adequate patient selection through strict inclusion and exclusion criteria. Patients over 40 years with prostate volume above 30 cm^3, with LUTS refractory to medical therapy for at least 6 months are selected for PAE, as are those patients who do not want to undergo medical or other more invasive surgical prostate therapies [3]. Patients under acute urinary retention due to BPO refractory to conservative management are also candidates for PAE. Patients without significant LUTS, with prostate cancer, with large (>5 cm) bladder diverticula or stone, bladder dysfunction, urinary tract infection or chronic renal failure are excluded. Patients should have evidence of BOO through, at least, non-invasive uroflowmetry to measure Qmax and post-void residual urine volume (PVR). In doubtful cases or for research purposes, invasive urodynamic studies should be performed before and after PAE, bearing in mind that these are examinations that induce significant patient discomfort. They can induce urinary tract infections or acute urinary retention in severely symptomatic patients.

PAE technique starts with pre-procedural planning [4]. We have performed 1150 PAE procedures from 2009–2016 and believe that pre-procedural CT angiography (CTA) of the pelvis is very important to define the arterial anatomy of pelvic and prostatic arteries (PAs) [5, 6]. Many centres are nowadays also performing PAE and prefer the use of intra-procedural cone-beam CT [7]. The use or not of pre-procedural CTA largely depends on physician/institutional preference. The use of pre-procedural MRI can also be of added value to exclude significant cancer and define prostate zonal anatomy. Either with pre-procedural CTA or intra-procedural conebeam CT it is essential to define the PA anatomy relevant for embolization. In our experience, pre-procedural CTA helps to decide which femoral artery or if both should be punctured, saving a lot of time during PAE in search of the 1–2 mm in size PAs amongst all internal iliac branches. We also exclude up to 2% of patients because PAE would be very difficult based on pre-procedural CTA. PAs can arise from aberrant obturator arteries outside the pelvis in up to 2% of patients [8], which is a variant that can lead to a huge amount of time and radiation wasted in search of PAs amongst the internal iliac branches if CTA is not performed before embolization.

PAE is performed on an outpatient basis, usually with a single femoral artery puncture under local anaesthesia [4]. We use a 5F Roberts uterine catheter (RUC, Cook Medical, Bloomington, IN) or a 5F Berenstein catheter to navigate both internal iliac arteries through a single femoral approach. The RUC catheter is a reversed catheter with a preformed Waltman loop. With the Berenstein catheter we use steam to bend the catheter 15–20 cm proximal to the tip to help reform the Waltman loop over the aortic bifurcation. When inside the internal iliac arteries, the steep ipsilateral anterior oblique projection (35–35°) with little caudal-cranial tilt (−10°) helps to separate and identify all the major branches, including the PAs. A standard digital subtraction angiography (DSA) or cone beam CT should be performed with the catheter tip in the proximal part of the anterior division of the internal iliac artery with the oblique projection. For DSA we use 6 mL at 3 mL/s, for cone beam-CT we use 10 mL at 1 mL/s with 1.5 s of delay. After this acquisition, the PAs are identified and selectively catheterized with 2.0–2.4F coaxial microcatheters. Our preferred microcatheter in recent times has been the Maestro (Merit Medical Systems Inc., South Jordan, UT, USA) that can be pre-shaped. We have used the Swan-neck shaped 2.4F Maestro even without a guide-wire (just the support from the 5F catheter) or with an 0.016″ guidewire for difficult catheterizations (GT, Terumo Interventional Systems, Tokyo, Japan or Tenor, Merit Medical Systems, Inc.).

The prostate has a dual arterial supply: feeding arteries for the central/cranial gland and for the peripheral/caudal gland. These two PAs may arise from a common trunk (one PA per pelvic side—60%) or have independent origins (two PAs per pelvic side—40%). In our experience most frequent PA origins are: (1) internal pudendal artery (35%); (2) superior vesical artery (20%); (3) directly from the anterior division of the internal iliac artery (15%); (4) obturator artery (10%) [5]. The remainder 20% are rare origins: prostato-rectal trunk, inferior or superior gluteal arteries and accessory pudendal arteries.

After identification and selective catheterization of the PAs cone-beam CT can be used to reassure correct target-embolization and identify possible anastomoses that may lead to non-target embolization of the bladder, rectum or penis (Fig. 6.2). Embolization of the PAs has been reported with the use of 50–350 μm PVA particles (Cook Medical, Bloomington, IN, USA; Boston Scientific Corp, Marlborough, Mass, USA), 300–500 μm spherical PVA (Beadblock, Biocompatibles International plc, Farnham, UK) and 100–300 and 300–500 μm tris-acryl gelatin microspheres (Embospheres, Merit Medical Systems, Inc.) to complete stasis, occlusion of all prostate branches and reflux to the main PA trunk.

6.3   Tips and Tricks

Starting with the access route, CTA can help to choose the best side to puncture the femoral artery and to decide between a short or long (more supportive) sheath in order to avoid tortuosity of iliac arteries and to ease the navigation of the equipment especially along the stiff and noncompliant ageing vessels. PAE has been reported to be successful from a transradial approach [9] and we have performed approximately 20 PAE procedures through a radial access. Even though being feasible, PAE can be even more challenging if adopting a radial access because of tortuosity of the aortic arch, common in patients older than 70 years, and lower support from the 5F catheter inside the pelvis. Existing catheters for radial access are 125 cm long, which allow reaching the internal iliac artery, but frequently fail to reach the PA ostium. The steep oblique projections used for PAE are also cumbersome for the operator when going through radial access as the X-ray C-arm can come very close to the operator. It is often useful to have the 5F catheter near the PA origin in order

Fig. 6.2 Cone-beam CT after bilateral selective PA catheterization with a microcatheter in a patient with a large prostate volume (185 cm³). An injection of 6 mL, at 0.5 mL/s was performed in each PA and overlay post-processing was performed to have both right and left acquisitions in the same image. (**a**) Coronal reformat, (**b**) axial reformat. In *red*, right PA; *blue*, left PA. Note the close proximity of the 5F catheter to the PA origin helping the microcatheter getting into the distal third of the PA trunk. Also note the marked tortuosity of the intra-prostatic arterial branches—corkscrew pattern

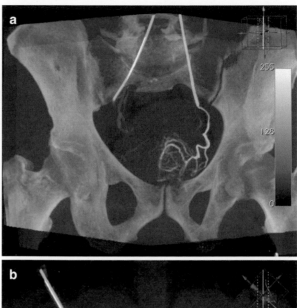

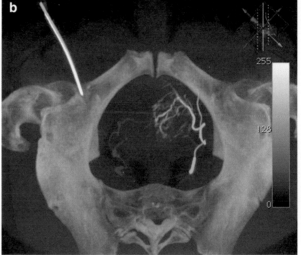

to help guide the microcatheter into the PA. From our experience, when using radial access, we always use 0.016″ guidewires to help guide the microcatheter into the PAs, while with the femoral approach we only need 0.016″ guidewires in approximately a third of procedures. However, in our experience, patient satisfaction is quite higher with radial access when compared to femoral, especially in those patients who frequently have to get out of bed to urinate after PAE.

More than 80% of PAs arise from the anterior division of the internal iliac artery. The superior vesical artery is one of the most common origins and is the first branch of the anterior division. Thus, when inside the internal iliac artery, the 5F catheter tip should be placed in the proximal part of the anterior division for a proper DSA run with the oblique views described above. This way, PAs can be identified and reached. We usually leave the 5F catheter tip near the PA origin and use its torque capability to help guide the microcatheter inside the PAs. We first try to use the swan-neck 2.4F Maestro without a guidewire, which we use only if we are not able to get into the PA. The superior vesical artery origin is usually the most difficult to selective catheterize. When possible, placing the 5F catheter tip in the superior vesical origin to guide the microcatheter down into the PA can be useful. Another option is to use 0.016″ guidewires to help direct the microcatheter down, distally to the vesical branches into the PA. If all that fails, coil embolization of the vesical branches can also be performed to help redirect flow of the embolics through reflux into the PA [4–6].

If two independent PAs are present, we embolize the central/cranial gland PA and leave the peripheral/caudal gland PA because BPH arises from the central gland. This way it is possible to induce selective central gland embolization and leave the peripheral prostate gland unembolized. If it is not possible to enter the central gland PA, we embolize the peripheral gland PA because there are frequent anastomoses between ipsilateral central/peripheral gland PAs that allow embolic migration from the peripheral to the central gland of the prostate. Peripheral gland PAs have variable amounts of anastomoses to the rectum, while central gland PAs have anastomoses to the bladder and penis.

After reaching the PA, a DSA or cone-beam CT should be performed prior to embolization to identify anastomoses that may lead to non-target embolization of the bladder, rectum or penis that may be present in up to 60% of PAs. Most of the times, these are small-sized distal branches that can be avoided with a careful and slow injection of the embolics. However, these anastomoses can have considerable sizes with higher risk of untargeted embolization. In these situations, coil block of these anastomoses should be performed prior to embolization to avoid embolic migration into prostate-surrounding organs. One specific type of these large anastomoses is the accessory pudendal artery that may provide arteries to both prostate and penis [4, 10–12].

6.4   PAE for Prostates Larger Than 100 cm³

The procedure is not necessarily easier in large prostates. Larger prostates do not correlate with larger PAs [5]. If a patient with a large prostate has duplicate PAs on both pelvic sides and is older and with atherosclerotic changes, he will have PAs smaller than those of a younger patient, with a 60 cm³ prostate but only one PA on each pelvic side. The number of PAs (and not prostate volume) correlates with PA trunk diameter [5]. However, the capsular and intra-prostatic branches of the PAs are larger in large prostates, making the typical corkscrew pattern of BPH nodule arteries easier to identify [5] (Fig. 6.2). PA origin, tortuosity and atherosclerosis are the most important predictors of technical success. Prostate volume was not different in patients with a successful bilateral PAE when compared with those with only unilateral PAE [13], thus prostate volume failed to correlate with technical success.

Regarding the potential role of prostate volume as predictor of clinical outcome after PAE there is conflicting evidence. We have shown that larger prostates had the same outcome as smaller ones and that prostate volume did not predict treatment outcome [14]. These findings were supported by others [15]; however, there is one study concluding that larger prostate volumes were associated with better outcomes after PAE [16]. We have also shown that MR-detected prostate infarction after PAE correlates with treatment outcome (Fig. 6.3), with larger areas of prostate ischemia associated with better clinical outcomes [14]. Prostate infarction had a stronger correlation with clinical outcome than prostate volume

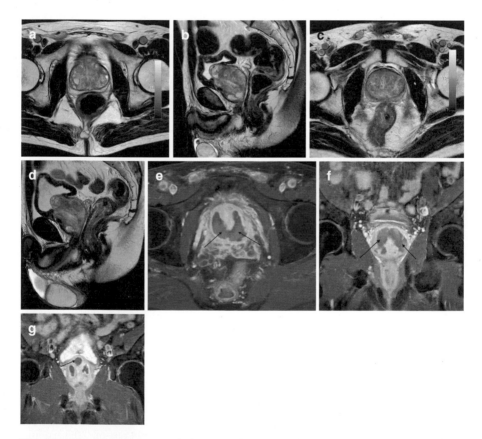

Fig. 6.3 MR of a large prostate before and after PAE. Axial (**a**) and sagital (**b**) T2 weighted images before embolization, prostate volume of 110 cm³. Axial (**c**) and sagital (**d**) T2 weighted images 18 days after embolization, prostate volume of 95 cm³—reduction of 14%. Axial (**e**) and coronal (**f, g**) T1 weighted images with fat-suppression after i.v. gadolineum injection. Large areas of ischemia in both lobes of the central gland are shown (*arrows*), also in the median lobe (**g**)

reduction after PAE [14]. However, prostate infarction correlated with prostate volume reduction and both with treatment outcome [14, 17]. PAE can induce significant prostate volume reduction (19.1%) in the various prostate gland anatomical zones with median lobe reductions of 26.2%, central gland of 18.8% and peripheral gland of 16.4% [17]. As PAE acts through central gland prostate-tissue destruction addressing the dynamic and static peri-urethral components of LUTS, it leads to fewer changes in the overall prostate gland size, similar to removing the content of an orange with an intact skin, leaving it devoid of content but with an intact outer surface. This may explain why some patients have significant clinical improvement after PAE and no prostate volume reduction, whereas others have significant prostate volume reductions without clinical improvement.

In prostates larger than 100 cm^3, PAE may be used as a preparatory step before prostate surgery for BPH patients. One to 3 months after PAE there is a substantial decrease in prostate volume that is sustained over time. This may allow a TURP procedure in some patients that would have to be treated with open surgery [18]. There are several published cohorts of BPH patients with large prostates treated by PAE [15, 16, 19–24], showing it to be safe and effective (Table 6.1). In these cohorts, mean prostate volume decreased from 110–140 to 71–91 cm^3 (31%–58%). Mean PSA reduction ranged from 5%–70%; mean IPSS reduction ranged from 13–20 points (49%–85%); mean QoL reduction ranged from 1.8–3.5 points (40%–73%) and mean Qmax increase ranged from 4–9.6 mL/s (40%–132%). The long-term results of PAE in 630 patients treated in our centre prove that PAE is a safe and effective technique with durable results [25]. We were able to collect data from 232 patients at 3 years and 103 patients at 4 years after PAE with a clinical success rate of 81%. At the time of writing there is only one randomized controlled trial from China comparing 57 patients who underwent TURP with 57 patients who underwent PAE [26]. At 24 months post-procedure, there were no significant differences in IPSS/QoL improvements or Qmax increase between the two groups. Clinical success rates were not significantly different between the two groups. However, prostate volume and PSA reductions were significantly larger in the TURP group. A retrospective analysis of a prospectively collected database using propensity score matching to compare 80 patients who underwent PAE to 80 patients who underwent open prostatectomy at 12 months follow-up, showed that surgery induced a significantly greater decrease in LUTS severity [27]. PSA reduction and Qmax increase were significantly better after surgery. PAE was associated with a significantly increased likelihood of persistent symptoms and persistent low Qmax but lower rate of adverse events with shorter hospitalization days and catheterization days. A recent meta-analysis of PAE [28] has shown that 12 months after PAE there is a mean prostate volume reduction of 31.31 cm^3 (P < 0.001), a mean PVR reduction of 85.54 mL (P < 0.001), a mean IPSS and QoL improvements of 20.39 points (P < 0.001) and 2.49 points (P < 0.001) with a mean Qmax increase of 5.39 mL/s (P < 0.001). PSA and IIEF remained unchanged. There were 32.93% of minor adverse events, the most common being rectalgia/dysuria (9.0%) and acute urinary retention (7.8%). There was no adverse effect on erectile function.

Table 6.1 Table summarizing existing literature on PAE for large prostate volumes

Ref. n.	Country	N. pts.	FU time, months	PV before, cm³	PV after, cm³	PV reduction, %	PSA reduction, ng/mL (%)	IPSS/QoL reduction, points (%)	Qmax increase, mL/s (%)
[15]	USA	36	6	139.4	N/A	N/A	N/A	12.9 (48.8)/3 (60)	N/A
[16]	China	64	12	129	74.5	58	3.4 (19)	14 (54)/3 (55)	6 (80)
[19]	Portugal	140	18	134.2	90	33	3.9 (44)	15 (60)/2.5 (55)	3.7 (40)
[20]	China	24	12	110	69	37	0.8 (16)	19.5 (72)/2.5 (55)	6 (50)
[21]	China	117	24	118	69	48	0.2 (5)	17 (65)/2 (40)	6 (71)
[22]	Brazil	35	3	135.1	91.9	32	4.7 (59)	15.6 (85)/1.8 (67)	8.1 (114)
[23]	Russia	88	12	129.3	71.2	45	1.6 (42)	13.6 (57)/N/A	9.6 (132)
[24]	USA	12	3	111.1	76.7	31	5.4 (70)	18.2 (76)/3.5 (73)	7.1 (116)

Ref. n. reference number, *N. pts.* number of patients, *FU* follow-up time, *PV* prostate volume, *PSA* prostate specific antigen, *IPSS* international prostate symptom score, *QoL* quality of life, *Qmax* peak urinary flowrate

In conclusion, PAE is becoming established as a therapeutic alternative to surgery with similar success in the improvement of LUTS and much fewer complications and morbidity. PAE can be a suitable option for patients with large prostates who do not want to undergo open prostatectomy or as a downsizing technique to allow endoscopic surgery.

References

1. Sun F, Crisóstomo V, Báez-Díaz C, Sánchez FM. Prostatic artery embolization (PAE) for symptomatic benign prostatic hyperplasia (BPH): part 2, insights into the technical rationale. Cardiovasc Intervent Radiol. 2016;39(2):161–9.
2. Oelke M, Bachmann A, Descazeaud A, et al.; European Association of Urology. EAU guidelines on the treatment and follow-up of non-neurogenic male lower urinary tract symptoms including benign prostatic obstruction. Eur Urol. 2013;64:118–40.
3. Pereira J, Bilhim T, Duarte M, Rio Tinto H, Fernandes L, Pisco JM. Patient selection and counseling before prostatic arterial embolization. Tech Vasc Interv Radiol. 2012;15:270–5.
4. Pisco JM, Pereira J, Rio Tinto H, Fernandes L, Bilhim T. How to perform prostatic arterial embolization. Tech Vasc Interv Radiol. 2012;15:286–9.
5. Bilhim T, Pisco JM, Rio Tinto H, et al. Prostatic arterial supply: anatomic and imaging findings relevant for selective arterial embolization. J Vasc Interv Radiol. 2012;23:1403–15.
6. Bilhim T, Rio Tinto H, Fernandes L, Pisco JM. Radiological anatomy of prostatic arteries. Tech Vasc Interv Radiol. 2012;15:276–85.
7. Bagla S, Rholl KS, Sterling KM, et al. Utility of cone-beam CT imaging in prostatic artery embolization. J Vasc Interv Radiol. 2013;24(11):1603–7.
8. Bilhim T, Pisco J, Campos Pinheiro L, Rio Tinto H, Fernandes L, Pereira JA. The role of accessory obturator arteries in prostatic arterial embolization. J Vasc Interv Radiol. 2014;25:875–9.
9. Isaacson AJ, Fischman AM, Burke CT. Technical feasibility of prostatic artery embolization from a transradial approach. AJR Am J Roentgenol. 2016;206(2):442–4.
10. Isaacson AJ, Bhalakia N, Burke CT. Coil embolization to redirect embolic flow during prostatic artery embolization. J Vasc Interv Radiol. 2015;26:768–70.
11. Amouyal G, Chague P, Pellerin O, et al. Safety and efficacy of occlusion of large extra-prostatic anastomoses during prostatic artery embolization for symptomatic BPH. Cardiovasc Intervent Radiol. 2016 Sep;39(9):1245–55.
12. Kably I, Dupaix R. Prostatic artery embolization and the accessory pudendal artery. J Vasc Interv Radiol. 2016;27(8):1266–8.
13. Bilhim T, Pisco J, Rio Tinto H, et al. Unilateral versus bilateral prostatic arterial embolization for lower urinary tract symptoms in patients with prostate enlargement. Cardiovasc Intervent Radiol. 2013 Apr;36(2):403–11.
14. Bilhim T, Pisco J, Pereira JA, et al. Predictors of clinical outcome after prostate artery embolization with spherical and nonspherical polyvinyl alcohol particles in patients with benign prostatic hyperplasia. Radiology. 2016 Oct;281(1):289–300.
15. Bagla S, Smirniotopoulos JB, Orlando JC, van Breda A, Vadlamudi V. Comparative analysis of prostate volume as a predictor of outcome in prostate artery embolization. J Vasc Interv Radiol. 2015;26(12):1832–8.
16. Wang M, Guo L, Duan F, et al. Prostatic arterial embolization for the treatment of lower urinary tract symptoms caused by benign prostatic hyperplasia: a comparative study of medium- and large-volume prostates. BJU Int. 2016;117(1):155–64.
17. Lin YT, Amouyal G, Correas JM, et al. Can prostatic arterial embolisation (PAE) reduce the volume of the peripheral zone? MRI evaluation of zonal anatomy and infarction after PAE. Eur Radiol. 2016;26(10):3466–73.

18. Nejmark AI, Nejmark BA, Tachalov MA, Arzamascev DD, Torbik DV. Superselective prostatic artery embolization as a preparatory step before TURP in the treatment of benign prostatic hyperplasia in patients with large prostates [in Russian]. Urologiia. 2015;(2):60–62, 64.
19. Pisco J, Bilhim T, Pinheiro LC, et al. Prostate embolization as an alternative to open surgery in patients with large prostate and moderate to severe lower urinary tract symptoms. Tech Vasc Interv Radiol. 2016;27:700–8.
20. Li Q, Duan F, Wang MQ, Zhang GD, Yuan K. Prostatic arterial embolization with small sized particles for the treatment of lower urinary tract symptoms due to large benign prostatic hyperplasia: preliminary results. Chin Med J. 2015;128(15):2072–7.
21. Wang MQ, Guo LP, Zhang GD, et al. Prostatic arterial embolization for the treatment of lower urinary tract symptoms due to large (>80 mL) benign prostatic hyperplasia: results of mid-term follow-up from Chinese population. BMC Urol. 2015;15:33.
22. de Assis AM, Moreira AM, de Paula Rodrigues VC, et al. Prostatic artery embolization for treatment of benign prostatic hyperplasia in patients with prostates > 90 g: a prospective single-center study. J Vasc Interv Radiol. 2015;26(1):87–93.
23. Kurbatov D, Russo GI, Lepetukhin A, et al. Prostatic artery embolization for prostate volume greater than 80 cm^3: results from a single-center prospective study. Urology. 2014;84(2):400–4.
24. Isaacson AJ, Raynor MC, Yu H, Burke CT. prostatic artery embolization using embosphere microspheres for prostates measuring 80-150 cm(3): early results from a US trial. J Vasc Interv Radiol. 2016;27(5):709–14.
25. Pisco JM, Bilhim T, Pinheiro LC, et al. Medium- and long-term outcome of prostate artery embolization for patients with benign prostatic hyperplasia: results in 630 patients. J Vasc Interv Radiol. 2016;27(8):1115–22.
26. Gao YA, Huang Y, Zhang R, et al. Benign prostatic hyperplasia: prostatic arterial embolization versus transurethral resection of the prostate--a prospective, randomized, and controlled clinical trial. Radiology. 2014;270(3):920–8.
27. Russo GI, Kurbatov D, Sansalone S, et al. Prostatic arterial embolization vs open prostatectomy: a 1-year matched-pair analysis of functional outcomes and morbidities. Urology. 2015;86(2):343–8.
28. Uflacker A, Haskal ZJ, Bilhim T, Patrie J, Huber T, Pisco JM. Meta-analysis of prostatic artery embolization for benign prostatic hyperplasia. J Vasc Interv Radiol. 2016. pii: S1051-0443(16)30439-0. doi: 10.1016/j.jvir.2016.08.004.

Chapter 7
Surgical Treatment: Enucleation of the Prostate

Rick Catterwell, Rick Popert, and Ben Challacombe

7.1 Introduction

Holmium laser enucleation of the prostate (HoLEP) is a trans-urethral technique for bladder outflow obstruction with a history and evidence base spanning over two decades. During this time enucleation has benefited from continued advances in energy technologies, improved availability of these energy sources and evolution of the surgical technique. The method has been standardised with retrograde enucleation of the prostate adenoma following its division into two or three anatomical lobes followed by mechanical morcellation of enucleated tissue. In the management of the large obstructive prostate, enucleation provides the benefits of endoscopic approaches while maintaining the anatomical considerations of open surgery.

The expanding transition zone adenoma in benign prostatic hyperplasia (BPH) results in a defined tissue plane between the adenoma and peripheral zone [2]. With laser incision and manipulation by the beak of the resectoscope the adenoma is dissected away from the peripheral zone. The enucleated tissue is dissected free into the bladder and then removed piecemeal from the bladder with a morcellation device. The utilization of the anatomical plane results in the removal of adenoma volume comparable to open/Millin's prostatectomy and facilitates favorable haemostasis. As laser enucleation is undertaken with saline irrigation and avoids dissection into prostatic venous channels the risk of post-resection absorption syndrome is negligible and there is thus no limit to the size of prostate than can be approached and HoLEP is a therefore an excellent option for surgical management of prostates greater than 100 cc [3, 4].

R. Catterwell (✉)
Guy's & St Thomas' Trust, London, UK

King's College Hospital, London, UK
e-mail: Rick.catterwell@gmail.com

R. Popert • B. Challacombe
Guy's & St Thomas' Trust, London, UK
e-mail: Rick.Popert@gstt.nhs.uk; benchallacombe@doctors.org.uk

© Springer International Publishing AG 2018
V. Kasivisvanathan, B. Challacombe (eds.), *The Big Prostate*,
https://doi.org/10.1007/978-3-319-64704-3_7

Table 7.1 Main advantages and limitations of holmium laser enucleation of the prostate compared to conventional transurethral resection of the prostate

Advantages	Limitations
Appropriate for all prostate sizes	Shallow/prolonged learning curve
Large glands can be completed in single surgery	Specific equipment required
Extremely low risk of post resection dilution syndrome	Technique unique to enucleation
Anti-coagulation not contra-indicated	Perceived risks of morcellation
Tissue removal equivalent to open prostatectomy	
Improved haemostasis	
Reduced length of hospital stay	

Based on all available evidence, HoLEP offers patients a safe, more efficient, and at least equally efficacious, if not more efficacious, treatment for BPH related LUTS when compared to other standard surgical therapies. These benefits have been consistently demonstrated in randomized controlled trials comparing HoLEP to TURP (see Table 7.1) and open prostatectomy [4–7]. Limited studies have been favourable for HoLEP compared to alternative laser treatments for BPH in regards to feasibility and durability with equivocal efficacy [8]. The result has been the emergence of laser enucleation of the prostate as the potential new gold standard for treating the symptomatic large prostate [9].

7.2 Patient Selection

The wide scope of patients appropriate for treatment with enucleation is an advantage of this technique. Patients with symptomatic bladder outlet obstruction (BOO) due to BPH are appropriate regardless of prostate size [10]. Larger sized glands have a tendency for a more defined plane between adenoma and peripheral zone aiding enucleation. From an anaesthetic standpoint HoLEP generally requires a general anaesthetic and can last up to three hours in men with the largest glands. Thus suitable men will need to be able to be anaesthetized for this length of time. Postoperative incontinence has previously been a worry in the adoption of HoLEP and requires specific mentoring to optimize enucleation techniques at the apex. In addition the cohort of men undergoing HoLEP are often those with the largest glands whose external sphincters may have been inactive for a long time and will thus require focused post-operative pelvic floor muscle training to optimize outcomes.

In contrast to embolization or vaporization techniques the anatomical configuration of the prostate is irrelevant and glands up to 500 cc in size have been successfully treated. Holmium laser enucleation is particularly suitable for the enlarged, intra-vesical median lobe where enucleation is effective and precise with minimal risk of injury to the trigone and ureteric orifices [2].

With the advantages of reduced fluid absorption, enhanced haemostasis, the use of saline irrigation and subsequent lack of post resection hyponatraemia syndrome there is reduced peri-operative cardio-vascular stress [3]. Although preference is for cessation of anti-coagulants prior to surgery the improved haemostatic properties of HoLEP have widened the scope in relation to patients where ceasing anti-coagulants is contra-indicated. HoLEP has been performed in patients on continued warfarin, clopidogrel or new generation anti-coagulant therapy (DOAC) [11, 12].

The presence of chronic urinary retention with confirmed detrusor under-activity is particularly suitable for enucleation. Likely due to the larger prostatic channel formation HoLEP has been demonstrated to have favorable spontaneous voiding rates and reduced post void residual volumes in independent trials and in comparison with photoselective vaporization of the prostate [13].

Pre-operative assessment should include urine microscopy and culture with surgery delayed for treatment of any active infection [14]. Symptomatology (IPSS) scores, voiding studies and PSA measurement allow pre- and post treatment evaluation. Estimation of prostate size with MRI or ultrasound is essential to advise patients, anaesthetists and for operating scheduling. Flexible cystoscopy is indicated if symptomatology or voiding flow studies suggest urethral stricture. Treatment of any urethral stricture disease and an observed period of stabilization of at least 6 months is recommended prior to enucleation.

7.3 Equipment

Enucleation of the prostate and subsequent extraction of the enucleated tissue from the bladder requires several specific equipment considerations. A 26F continuous flow sheath is combined with a laser resectoscope either with a dedicated laser channel facilitating thumb controlled advancement of the laser fibre (Fig. 7.1b) or a laser inner sheath with a stabilizing guide. If the latter is used the fibre is passed through a ureteric catheter and interlink port (Fig. 7.1a) which is passed through the stabilizing circular ring with in the inner lumen of the inner sheath.

7.3.1 Laser

The Holmium:YAG laser is a pulsed solid state laser, with a wavelength of 2140 nm that acts through a predominately photothermal mechanism. On soft tissue this laser has an absorption depth of only 0.4 mm with tissue ablated faster than heat is conducted into surrounding tissue. As a result the holmium laser is ideal for cleanly ablating without charring or overheating adjacent tissue. In contrast to the KTP 'Greenlight" laser, the Holmium wavelength is highly absorbed by saline

Fig. 7.1 Laser
resectoscopes used in
holmium laser enucleation
of the prostate. (**a**)
Continuous flow sheath
combined with a laser
resectoscope that has a
laser inner sheath with a
stabilizing guide. (**b**)
Continuous flow sheath
combined with a laser
resectoscope that a
dedicated laser channel
facilitating thumb
controlled advancement of
the laser fibre

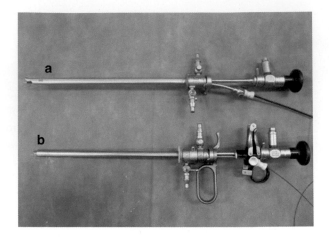

or water. With separation from fibre to tissue of 4 mm, less than 1% of energy
reaches the tissue, greatly reducing risk of unintended vaporization of distant tissue
such as the posterior bladder wall or trigone.

In the historical development of laser surgery for BPH early techniques combined the use of Holmium:YAG (Yttrium-Aluminium-Garnet) and neodymium
(Nd:YAG) lasers. The combination endoscopic laser ablation of the prostate
(CELAP) utilized the cutting properties of the Ho:YAG laser and the coagulation
properties of the Nd:YAG laser. This technique was complicated by significant
indwelling catheter times post operatively, ranging from 4.1 to 7.1 days. In addition
many patients had significant irritative voiding symptoms and subsequent episodes
of urinary retention.

With advances in technique and technology it became evident at sufficient power
the Holmium laser had adequate haemostatic effects. By the late 1990s Kabalin had
demonstrated in canine and human studies that haemostatic vaporization of prostate
tissue was achieved with the Holmium laser alone using high power ranges of
50–80 W. Its localized coagulation effect 'seals' the tissue and provides hemostasis
superior to electrocautery instruments without producing deeper thermal injury
associated with Nd:YAG laser.

As a tissue vaporizing instrument the Holmium laser is not efficient. Initial application of this laser for a purely vaporizing technique resulted in the holmium laser
ablation of the prostate, termed HoLAP. This resulted in less necrosis of adjacent
tissue and irritative symptoms compared with the combination procedures using the
Nd:YAG laser. Although irritative symptoms and sloughing were reduced operative
times were prolonged and the technique therefore restricted to small prostates or as
part of a HoLEP learning process.

Gilling et al. in 1996 were the first to describe a holmium laser resection of the prostate. This technique was the first to utilize the cutting properties of the holmium laser to detach large sections of adenoma tissue. The absence of post-operative dilutional hyponatraemia and transfusion requirements were reproduced in numerous published series over multiple centers.

Over the subsequent two decades the application of high powered holmium lasers as a cutting and coagulating tool have been further advanced with the ability to adjust the laser pulse width. The same energy output delivered in shorter pulse duration enhances the lasers' cutting properties. As a result tissue planes are more easily demonstrated with minimal charring of adjacent tissue. Conversely with the energy delivered over wide pulse duration an increase in penetration and width of effect results in an enlarged heat affected zone and increased heat conduction time. This has a clinical effect of improving the coagulation ability of the holmium laser. Although not essential for the procedure, dual setting, high energy, holmium laser units up to 120 W have become increasing popular for enucleation.

Various authors advocate different laser settings. Expert opinion varies with a frequency between 30–50 Hz and energy of 1.8–2.0 J [2, 14]. There is a paucity of published literature advocating wide pulse width settings on dual setting units with manufacturers' recommendations suggesting reduced energy (1.2–1.6 J) with similar frequency (30–40 Hz).

7.3.2   Morcellation

Initial descriptions of Holmium resection of the prostate by Gilling and Fraundorfer involved the resection of tailored fragments of prostate that could be removed with the aid of either a modified resectoscope loop or Ellik evacuator [15]. The addition of mechanical morcellation of resected prostatic tissue, originally via a supra-pubic tract and later trans-urethrally, facilitated complete enucleation of the prostate. Holmium Laser Enucleation of the Prostate was thus truly conceived by Gilling and Fraundorfer with the addition of mechanical morcellation [16].

The mechanical morcellator consists of a hand-piece with 5-mm reciprocating blades (Fig. 7.3). Control is via a multiple staged foot control, which engages progressively from zero suction, suction, suction with low speed blade reciprocation and suction with high-speed blade reciprocation. This is passed down a long nephroscope which is connected to the 26F outer sheath by a specific adapter. Double inflow irrigation is recommended to ensure bladder distention during morcellation thus reducing the risk of bladder injury.

7.4 Technique

Enucleation can be performed with general or spinal anaesthesia although many units prefer a general anaesthetic to reduce the chance of excessive movement, particularly during the morcellation phase of the procedure. Haemostasis can be challenging if adequate systolic blood pressure control is not achieved.

The patient is positioned in lithotomy with adequate hip flexion and abduction to facilitate the range of scope manipulation required. Single dose broad-spectrum prophylactic antibiotics and mechanical DVT prevention are recommended.

7.4.1 Enucleation

A routine cystoscopy is performed to exclude any concomitant pathology such as urethral stricture, bladder calculi or bladder lesion. In the presence of urethral stricture enucleation should be aborted until the stricture is treated and sufficiently followed up without recurrence. Bladder calculi are easily managed with the holmium laser prior to commencing the enucleation. Dilatation of the anterior urethral to 30F with serial sounds is then performed to allow easy passage of the 26F continuous flow resectoscope.

Bilateral bladder neck incisions are then made, extending from bladder neck to verumontanum. These incisions are extended to the level of the surgical capsule, a clearly identified smooth fibrous layer (Fig. 7.2). If no median lobe is pres-

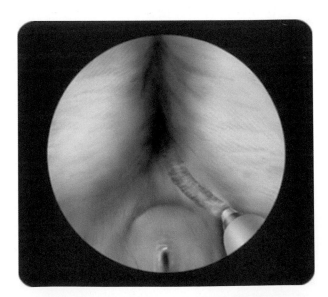

Fig. 7.2 Bilateral bladder neck incisions are extended to the level of the surgical capsule, a clearly identified smooth fibrous layer

ent, a single incision can be made at the 6 o'clock position. With each encountered bleeding vessel haemostasis is achieved via either defocusing the laser by retracting it from the tissue slightly or utilizing the broad pulse width setting with a dual setting laser unit.

The bladder neck incisions are sculpted medial along their course from the bladder neck to the verumontanum leaving a midline strip of tissue attaching the median lobe to the surgical capsule (Fig. 7.3). Commencing from just proximal to the veru-

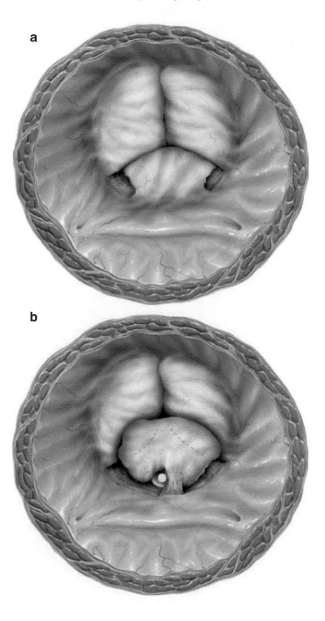

a

b

Fig. 7.3 The bladder neck incisions are sculpted medial along their course from the bladder neck to the verumontanum leaving a midline strip of tissue attaching the median lobe to the surgical capsule

montanum the bladder neck incisions are connected. The beak of the resectoscope is used to elevate the median lobe to facilitate demonstration of the remaining fibres connecting the median lobe to the capsule which are divided (Fig. 7.4). By working from side to side, from each medialized bladder neck incision, the strip of remaining tissue is divided and the median lobe is enucleated. The location of the ureteric orifices should be closely monitored during the final manipulation of the enucleation at the bladder neck to avoid injury.

Enucleation of the lateral lobes begins with identification of the surgical plane at the level of the verumontanum. The surgical plane is expanded using a combination of scope manipulation and laser energy laterally to define the apex. The plane is also advanced proximally (Fig. 7.5).

Once the apex has been defined to the 2 o'clock position attention moves to the anterior prostate. A midline incision anteriorly is made from bladder neck back to the level of the verumontanum. The bladder neck mucosa is sculpted laterally from this incision and the incision is deepened and extended laterally and distally exposing the surgical plane from above (Fig. 7.6).

The upper and lower incisions are connected at the apex by laser incision of the joining mucosal bridge and the lateral lobe is enucleated in the capsular plane, working from the upper to lower incisions in a manner analogous to the median lobe enucleation (Fig. 7.7).

Meticulous consideration of haemostasis should be undertaken prior to morcellation as optimal vision is needed before commencing morcellation and it is inefficient to go back to using the laser after this point.

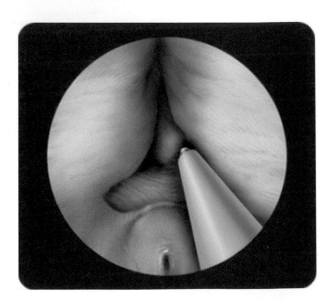

Fig. 7.4 The beak of the resectoscope is used to elevate the median lobe to facilitate demonstration of the remaining fibres connecting the median lobe to the capsule which are divided

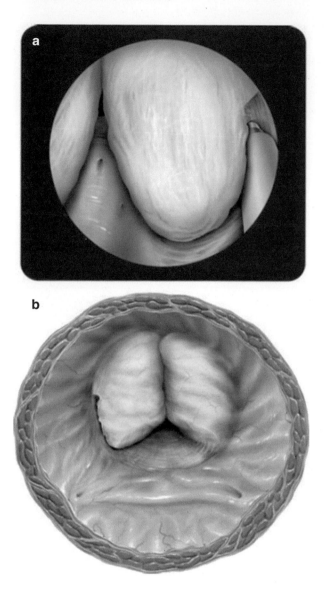

Fig. 7.5 Enucleation of the lateral lobes begins with identification of the surgical plane at the level of the verumontanum. The surgical plane is expanded using a combination of scope manipulation and laser energy laterally to define the apex. The plane is also advanced proximally

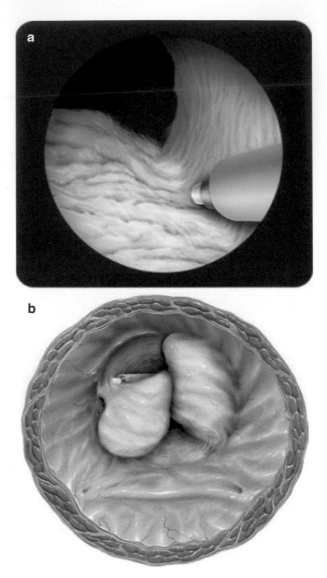

Fig. 7.6 Once the apex has been defined to the 2 o'clock position attention moves to the anterior prostate. A midline incision anteriorly is made from bladder neck back to the level of the verumontanum. The bladder neck mucosa is sculpted laterally from this incision and the incision is deepened and extended laterally and distally exposing the surgical plane from above

Fig. 7.7 The upper and lower incisions are connected at the apex by laser incision of the joining mucosal bridge and the lateral lobe is enucleated in the capsular plane, working from the upper to lower incisions in a manner analogous to the median lobe enucleation

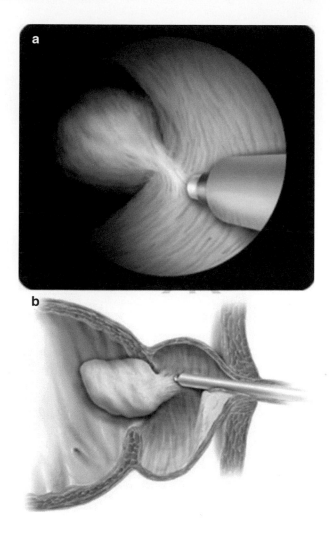

7.4.2   Morcellation

To facilitate morcellation the continuous flow inner sheath is replaced with a long, 'off-set' nephroscope and adaptor. Avoiding bladder decompression during this change of instruments can aid vision. The bladder is fully distended and the 5 mm bladed morcellator is introduced down the nephroscope working channel. Suction is activated by the foot pedal, allowing prostate fragments to be engaged and positioned at the bladder neck with the morcellator jaws directed upwards and away from the trigone (Fig. 7.8). Small fragments, resistant to morcellation, are removed with either a grasping loop or Ellik evacuator.

Fig. 7.8 The bladder is fully distended and the 5 mm bladed morcellator is introduced down the nephroscope working channel. Suction is activated by the foot pedal, allowing prostate fragments to be engaged and positioned at the bladder neck with the morcellator jaws directed upwards and away from the trigone

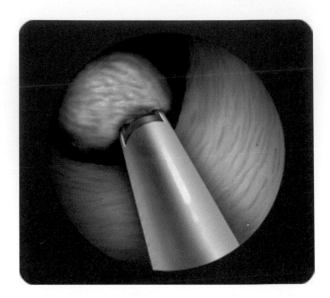

During early series morcellation was associated with a high incidence of bladder mucosal injury. Maintenance of irrigating fluid during morcellation should be fastidious. A simple modification of technique making use of double irrigation has virtually eliminated this complication [17]. Irrigation flows through both the 'normal inflow' via the nephroscope and also via the 'normal out flow' from the outer 26F sheath. Actual outflow is from the morcellator hand piece only. This double inflow maintains bladder distention, keeping the mucosa away from the morcellator blades.

7.5   Comparison

Over the past two decades HoLEP has had a massive impact on the management of men with obstructive large prostates [9]. Previously men with adenomas too large for endoscopic resection (>100 cc) were directed towards open prostatectomy (OP). Favorable results have been consistently demonstrated for HoLEP compared to OP in relation to transfusion rates, length of hospitalization and catheterization [6, 7, 18]. More recently alternative surgical techniques to HoLEP have been suggested although evidence in larger prostates is sparse with concerns regarding feasibility and durability in large glands [8, 19].

There is robust evidence demonstrating HoLEP has favorable outcomes regardless of prostate size. Kuntz, et al. [10] detail a prospective series of 389 patients stratified by prostate size (<40, 40–79 and >80 g). 121 (31.5%) of the cohort had prostates greater than 80 g (range 80–260 g). They found no differences in perioperative morbidity and postoperative micturition improvement across the cohorts. No patients required blood transfusion. There was no significant difference in duration of catheterization or admission. Similarly, Lingeman et al. [20] retrospectively reviewed 507 patients stratified into three groups based on preoperative volume measurements. They found no significant difference in hospital stay, catheterization time, post-operative AUA-SS, and post-operative Q max among the three groups.

7.5.1 HoLEP vs. OP

Several randomized control trials (RCTs) have directly compared HoLEP and OP outcomes. Montorsi et al. [6] performed a randomized prospective trial comparing HoLEP and OP in 80 patients with obstructive symptoms and estimated prostate volumes >70 g. They demonstrated significantly lower transfusion rate (4% vs. 17.9%), quicker time to removal of catheter (1.5 vs. 4.1 days) and shorter length of hospitalization (2.7 vs. 5.4 days) in favor of HoLEP. Functional results for HoLEP were similar to OP over the 2-year follow-up period. Moody and Lingeman, et al. [15] retrospectively compared HoLEP to OP in prostates >100 g and found that patients who underwent HoLEP benefitted from a minimal change in postoperative hemoglobin (1.3 vs. 2.9 g/dL) and shorter length of stay (2.1 vs. 6.1 days) despite a greater amount of adenoma resected (151 vs. 106 g). Symptom score improvement was equivalent between groups.

7.5.2 HoLEP vs. PVP

Greenlight photo vaporization of the prostate (PVP) is the most well established laser alternative to TURP and HoLEP. It utilizes the coupling of a Nd:YAG laser with a potassium-titanyl-phosphate (KTP) crystal resulting in a halving of the laser wavelength to 532 nm. This visible laser has substantially different laser-tissue interaction properties than the uncoupled Nd:YAG laser. The KTP laser beam is highly absorbed by hemoglobin inside prostatic tissue resulting in rapid photothermal vaporization of heated intracellular water and efficient vaporization of prostatic adenoma. The coagulation zone thickness (1-2 mm) is relatively shallow compared to the Nd:YAG laser (7 mm) reducing coagulation necrosis associated post-operative dysuria and sloughing [21]. Less favorably the laser beam is fully transmitted through irrigation fluid with risk of distant site injury to the bladder wall especially during median lobe vaporization.

Technological advances in the power output from KTP lasers have improved the rate of vaporization and facilitated treatment of larger adenomas [19, 21]. Improvement from the initially underpowered 80 W KTP laser to the high-powered 120 W and now 180 W models has undoubtedly improved outcomes. As a result comparison is complicated and long term follow up regarding the durability of PVP treatment in large glands is sparse.

Few RCTs comparing HoLEP and PVP have been performed. Elmansy et al. [8] reported the first randomized controlled clinical trial comparing HoLEP to PVP using a 120 W KTP laser and included cohorts with large prostates of comparable volumes (91.3 g vs. 89.3 g). There was no significant difference in IPSS, quality of life, or sexual function at one year. The HoLEP cohort had a significantly higher maximal flow rate and lower post void residual. Intra-operatively 22% of PVP patients required conversion to either HoLEP or TURP due bleeding that was uncontrollable with the PVP laser. In the converted cases, a mean of 46 g of further prostate tissue was removed by HoLEP or TURP.

An initial multicenter RCT comparing HoLEP and PVP with a 180 W KTP laser outcomes has demonstrated no difference in morbidity rates, re-intervention rates or length of hospital stay. Despite prostate size reduction being greater in the HoLEP cohort there was no significant difference in symptoms scores between the two groups to the study end point of 12 months [19].

7.5.3   Durability

The durability of HoLEP results has been extensively studied and is a major strength of the technique. Several studies have followed HoLEP patients for between 5 and 10 years, with a re-operation rate of less than 1%. Gilling et al. [22] reported in a RCT of HoLEP vs. TURP a reoperation rate of zero vs. 18% at 7 years in the HoLEP and TURP cohorts respectively. Kuntz [18] et al. also reported a reoperation rate of zero at 5 years for men with prostates >100 g who underwent HoLEP.

7.6   Limitations of HoLEP and Learning Curve

Despite its many potential advantages there is little doubt that the HoLEP procedure has a significant learning curve and that one is certainly better and more efficient after 200 procedures than one was after 50. The learning curve is therefore not steep but shallow as it takes many cases to become truly proficient. In terms of the learning curve for safety and enucleation efficiency (enucleated weight/enucleation time) and morcellation efficiency this seems to be around 40–60 cases for larger prostates [23] but may be only 25 cases in smaller glands [24].

Initial concerns about damage to the external sphincter and morcellation injury to the bladder during the learning period have reduced as the surgical technique has been standardised and modern dedicated equipment has evolved. It has been shown that older men with larger prostates are more vulnerable to post operative incontinence and also that mentored surgeons caused less incontinence than those learning in isolation [25]. There are now good educational videos available on line with dedicated courses at most major urological meetings. However, without an experienced mentor and a dedicated team approach those attempting HoLEP are not always universally successful in making the procedure part of their standard repertoire [26]. Learning should therefore be carefully planned with a gradual increase in case complexity/prostate size as experience increases [27].

7.7 HoLEP and Prostate Cancer Active Surveillance in the Large Prostate

Rising prostate specific antigen in men with lower urinary tract symptoms can be a cause of concern, especially for patients on active surveillance for low-risk prostate cancer. PSA often reflects transition zone hyperplasia in large prostates even with co-existing low risk prostate cancer. Many men have already undergone a prostatic biopsy and are concerned about prostate cancer risk. Popert et al. in retrospective study of 30 patients undergoing HoLEP on a background of low risk prostate cancer on active surveillance demonstrated a median reduction in PSA of 85% with a median resection of 94 g [28]. The reduction in PSA has been demonstrated to highly correlate to the amount of prostatic tissue removed [20] and provide huge reassurance to this cohort of men.

Removal of the transition zone via HoLEP significantly reduces PSA resulting in PSA becoming more cancer specific. Most post HoLEP PSA levels are in the 1–2 μg/L range and thus any significant rise above this new baseline or failure of the PSA to drop post HoLEP is likely to signify significant prostate cancer. These men need education on their new post HoLEP PSA levels as do their primary care providers in order to react to any future rise. With prostate cancer progression requiring active treatment, reduction in gland size with HoLEP may facilitate prostate cancer treatment options normally precluded by gland volume such as brachytherapy or external beam radiation [28].

7.8 Conclusion

There have been many procedures proposed as alternatives to TURP for the surgical treatment of BOO secondary to BPH. With advancing life expectancy the incidence of prostatic enlargement beyond what was traditionally feasible for endoscopic resection is increasing.

The ideal procedure to manage both the large obstructing prostate is minimally invasive, effective, durable and associated with low morbidity and complication rates. Ideally it would be a technique that is applicable to all prostate sizes and anatomical configurations. The evidence base in support of HoLEP is more extensive than that for any other alternative. HoLEP is at least as effective as other surgical therapies, including TURP, OP and other laser modalities, with fewer complications, shorter hospital stays, and decreased catheter time. In the larger gland, including those greater than 100 cc, HoLEP stands alone as the gold standard. Morbidity, complication and reoperation rates appear lower than alternatives with durability confirmed over 10 years of follow up.

The HoLEP procedure has now passed the tests of safety, efficacy, and durability. It is a strong contender for the new gold standard for endoscopic BPH surgery in prostates of all sizes especially for larger glands. The challenge for HoLEP is continued expansion of its clinical application, to shed perceptions of difficulties in adopting the technique via improved mentoring and teaching during structured urological training.

References

1. Gilling PJKK, Das AK, Thompson DFM. Holmium laser enucleation of the prostate (HoLEP) combined with transurethral tissue morcellation: an update on the early clinical experience. J Endourol. 1998;12:457–9.
2. Gilling PJ. Surgical atlas—Holmium Laser Enucleation of the Prostate (HoLEP). BJU Int. 2008;101:131–42.
3. Shah HNKV, Hegde S, et al. Evaluation of fluid absorption during holmium laser enucleation of prostate by breath ethanol technique. J Urol. 2006;175:537–40.
4. Tan AHHGP, Kennett KM, Frampton C, Westenberg AM, Fraundorfer MR. A randomized trial comparing holmium laser enucleation of the prostate with transurethral resection of the prostate for the treatment of bladder outlet obstruction secondary to benign prostatic hyperplasia in large glands (40–200 grams). J Urol. 2003;170:1270–4.
5. Montorsi FNR, Salonia A, et al. Holmium laser enucleation versus transurethral resection of the prostate: results from a 2-center prospective randomized trial in patients with obstructive benign prostatic hyperplasia. J Urol. 2004;172:1926–9.
6. Naspro RSN, Salonia A, et al. Holmium laser enucleation of the prostate versus open prostatectomy for prostates >70g: 24-month follow-up. Eur Urol. 2006;50:563–8.
7. Kuntz RMLK. Transurethral holmium enucleation versus transvesical open enucleation for prostate adenoma greater than 100 gm. A randomized prospective trial of 120 patients. J Urol. 2002;168:1465–9.
8. Elmansy HBA, Kotb A, Badawy H, Riad E, Emran A, Elhilali M. Holmium laser enucleation versus photoselective vaporization for prostatic adenoma greater than 60 ml: preliminary results of a prospective, randomized clinical trial. J Urol. 2012;188:216–21.
9. Vincent MWGP. HoLEP has come of age. World J Urol. 2015;33(4):487–93.
10. Kuntz RMLK, Ahyai S. Does perioperative outcome of transurethral holmium laser enucleation of the prostate depend on prostate size? J Endourol. 2004;18(2):183–8.
11. Elzayat E HE, Elhilali M. Holmium laser enucleation of the prostate in patients on anticoagulant therapy or with bleeding disorders. J Urol. 2006;175:1428–32.
12. Bishop CV, Liddell H, Ischia J, Paul E, Appu S, Frydenberg M, Pham T. Holmium laser enucleation of the prostate: comparison of immediate postoperative outcomes in patients with and without antithrombotic therapy. Curr Urol. 2013;7(1):28–33.
13. Raison NCB. Opening the flood gates: holmium laser enucleation is superior to photoselective vaporization of the prostate for the treatment of chronic urinary retention. BJU Int. 2015;115(2):178–9.
14. Kuo RL, Paterson RF, Kim SC, Siqueira TM Jr, Elhilali MM, Lingeman JE. Holmium Laser Enucleation of the Prostate (HoLEP): a technical update. World J Surg Oncol. 2003;1:6–7.
15. Gilling PJ, Cass CB, Cresswell MD, Malcolm AR, Fraundorfer MR. The use of the holmium laser in the treatment of benign prostatic hyperplasia. J Endourol. 1996;10:459–61.
16. Fraundorfer MRGP. Holmium: YAG laser enucleation of the prostate combined with mechanical morcellation: preliminary results. Eur Urol. 1998;33(1):69–72.
17. Cynk MH. Holmium laser enucleation of the prostate: a review of the clinical trial evidence. Ther Adv Urol. 2014;6(2):62–73. http://doi.org/10.1177/1756287213511509

18. Kuntz RMLK, Ahyai SA. Holmium laser enucleation of the prostate versus open prostatectomy for prostates greater than 100 grams: 5-year follow-up results of a randomised clinical trial. Eur Urol. 2008;53:160–6.
19. Elshal AMEM, El-Nahas AR, Shoma AM, Nabeeh A, Carrier S, Elhilali MM. GreenLight™ laser (XPS) photoselective vapo-enucleation versus holmium laser enucleation of the prostate for the treatment of symptomatic benign prostatic hyperplasia: a randomized controlled study. J Urol. 2015;193(3):927–34.
20. Humphreys MR, Miller NL, Handa SE, Terry C, Munch LC, Lingeman JE. Holmium laser enucleation of the prostate—outcomes independent of prostate size? J Urol. 2008;180(6):2431–5.
21. Sountoulides P, Tsakiris P. The evolution of the KTP laser vaporization of the prostate. Yonsei Med J. 2008;49(2):189–99.
22. Gilling PJWL, King CJ, Westenberg AM, Frampton CM, Fraundorfer MR. Long-term results of a randomized trial comparing holmium laser enucleation of the prostate and transurethral resection of the prostate: results at 7 years. BJU Int. 2012;109:408–11.
23. Brunckhorst O, Ahmed K, Nehikhare O, Marra G, Challacombe B, Popert R. Evaluation of the learning curve for holmium laser enucleation of the prostate using multiple outcome measures. Urology. 2015;86(4):824–9.
24. Jeong CW, Oh JK, Cho MC, Bae JB, Oh SJ. Enucleation ratio efficacy might be a better predictor to assess learning curve of holmium laser enucleation of the prostate. Int Braz J Urol. 2012;38(3):362–71; discussions 72.
25. Shigemura K, Tanaka K, Yamamichi F, Chiba K, Fujisawa M. Comparison of predictive factors for postoperative incontinence of holmium laser enucleation of the prostate by the surgeons' experience during learning curve. Int Neurourol J. 2016;20(1):59–68.
26. Robert G, Cornu JN, Fourmarier M, Saussine C, Descazeaud A, Azzouzi AR, et al. Multicentre prospective evaluation of the learning curve of holmium laser enucleation of the prostate (HoLEP). BJU Int. 2016;117(3):495–9.
27. Elshal AM, Nabeeh H, Eldemerdash Y, Mekkawy R, Laymon M, El-Assmy A, et al. Prospective assessment of learning curve of holmium laser enucleation of the prostate for treatment of benign prostatic hyperplasia using a multidimensional approach. J Urol. 2016;
28. Marra G NO, Samad, S, Kinsella J, Van Hemelrijck M, Ahmed K, Challacombe B, Popert R. Enucleation of the transition zone and the effect on PSA in patients with lower urinary tract symptoms. J Urol. 2015;193(4):e913.

Chapter 8
Surgical Treatment: Green Light Laser

Clarissa Martyn-Hemphill, Srinath Chandrasekera, and Gordon Muir

8.1   Introduction

Transurethral photoselective vaporization of the prostate (PVP) has evolved as an electrosurgical adaptation of the classical transurethral resection of the prostate (TURP) in the management of bladder outflow obstruction (BOO). Improvements in Light Amplification by Stimulated Emission of Radiation (laser) technology have shown potential for excellent haemostasis, a reduction in morbidity and good functional outcomes. The increasing role of PVP as a true 'day case' procedure has made it an attractive focus for clinicians and hospital managers in the age of healthcare economics.

The application of lasers in urology has been recognised and incorporated into the EAU and AUA guidelines in selected patients with BOO. TURP remains the transurethral standard for comparison, but in larger prostates, a prolonged resection time is invariably required. Historically, many surgeons would choose an open prostatectomy (OP) in this patient group to avoid the morbidity relating to bleeding and/or possible development of TUR syndrome.

This chapter will address the emerging utility, safety and efficacy profile of PVP as a valid alternative treatment of BOO in men with large prostates, including those over 100 mL, and the challenges that this modality presents.

C. Martyn-Hemphill (✉) • G. Muir
Kings College Hospital, London, UK
e-mail: cmartynhemphill@gmail.com; gordonhmuir@gmail.com

S. Chandrasekera
Professor of Urology, University of Sri Jayawardanapura, Colombo, Sri Lanka
e-mail: schandre@hotmail.com

© Springer International Publishing AG 2018   105
V. Kasivisvanathan, B. Challacombe (eds.), *The Big Prostate*,
https://doi.org/10.1007/978-3-319-64704-3_8

8.2   Mechanism of Action

Potassium-titanyl-phosphate (KTP) laser prostatectomy was first described by *Kuntzman* and colleagues in a comparative functional study against a Neodymium:Yttrium-Aluminum-Garnet (Nd:YAG) laser in canines in 1996 [1]. KTP vaporization was found to be significantly superior, with instantaneous reduction in prostate volume and spontaneous post-operative voiding. This was unlike the coagulative necrosis triggered by the Nd:YAG laser: which took weeks for the prostatic tissue to slough off and was often associated with storage symptoms.

GreenLight laser vaporisation differs in technique to laser enucleation of the prostate. Prostatic tissue is entirely vaporised, rather than enucleated and mechanically morcellated. The 532 nm wavelength generated by the KTP crystal falls within the visible green zone of the electromagnetic spectrum; hence 'GreenLight' laser. This accounts for its near exclusive absorption by haemoglobin, and not water; thus its enhanced ability to secure haemostasis within highly vascularised prostatic tissue [2].

The feasibility of the 80 W KTP PVP was subsequently trialled in humans (prostate volumes of 24–76 mL) with BPH by Malek et al. in 1998 [3]. This was replaced by the high-performance system (HPS) GreenLight 120 W (532 nm) laser which was introduced in 2006. GreenLight HPS used a Lithium Triborate (LBO) crystal in the place of KTP [4]. It has been further superseded by the 180 W GreenLight Xcelerated Performance System (XPS) in 2010 (American Medical Systems, Minnetonka, MI). Unlike earlier generations, the MoXy fibre within the XPS is a 750 nm side-firing laser with a 70° forward deflection. It also includes a steel-tipped cap and fibre cooling to prevent overheating and optimise fibre durability (i.e. one fibre per case). Compared to the HPS, the beam surface area is augmented from 0.28 to 0.44 mm^2 [5]. The laser is fired in a quasi-continuous wave laser rapid pulse to elicit vaporisation through a 23–26F cystoscope with normal saline irrigation fluid on continuous flow [6]. Compared to GreenLight HPS in prostate volumes of >80 mL, similar amounts of energy are used in significantly less time ($P = 0.001$) [7]. The ease at which an operative working channel can be created, reduces the risk of excess fluid absorption and dilutional hyponatraemia in these patients.

8.3   Operative Technique

GreenLight PVP can be performed under light general or regional anaesthesia; as there is no risk of TUR syndrome, even in massive prostates [8]; most experts avoid spinal anaesthesia. Unlike TURP, there is not always tissue for histopathological examination at the end of the procedure (transperineal biopsy is simple however if clinically indicated). The technique is non-contact (optimum fibre tissue distance = 1–2 mm). The pilot beam is used to guide the dissemination of energy evenly by a systematic "three-dimensional, sagittal, rotating and lateral motion of the fibre" [6]. An appropriate sweep speed is required to prevent carbonisation and ineffective ablation. Failure to do so may result in overheating and damage of the fibre and/or scope from heat reflection. The vaporisation results in vapour bubbles, which are carried away by the continuous flow setup with gravity inflow and outflow.

There is an increasing availability of validated computer simulation programmes to promote a sustained and standardised level of procedural excellence in GreenLight laser prostatectomies. Training and assessment of operative technique can be undertaken safely for small, medium and large glands (Figs. 8.1 and 8.2). The learning curve of proficiency for GreenLight prostatectomy builds upon fundamental principles of safe transurethral electrosurgical techniques and is comparably less technically challenging than HoLEP [9].

8.4   Adverse Events and Sexual Function

The search for alternative surgical modalities for BPH relates to the ongoing rate of morbidity associated with TURP. Teng et al. undertook a comparative systematic review and meta-analysis of RCTs and non-RCTs (n = 9) evaluating TURP and GreenLight laser PVP outcome data. Overall, the rates of bleeding (requiring

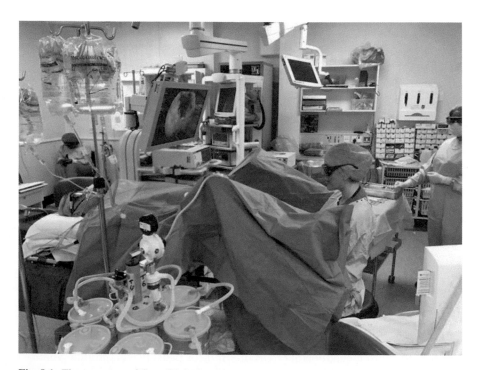

Fig. 8.1 Theatre set up of GreenLight Laser

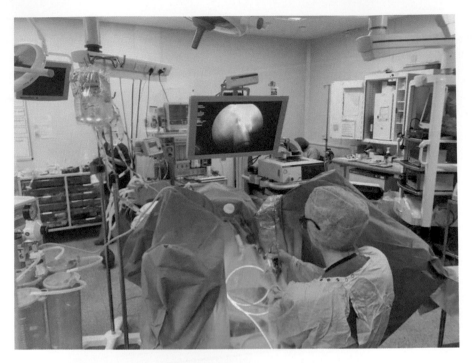

Fig. 8.2 Creating the working channel with GreenLight Laser intra-operatively

transfusion RR =5.88, 95% CI:1.92–18.3, $P = 0.002$) capsular perforation (RR = 9.28, 95%CI: 2.79–30.88, $P = 0.001$) and TUR syndrome (RR =5.31, 95% CI:1.18–23.94, $P = 0.003$) were shown to be considerably lower in the PVP groups than for those undergoing TURP [10].

Another recent meta-analysis identified six RCTs evaluating PVP with GreenLight HPS 120 W device against monopolar TURP (697 patients). Statistical significance was demonstrated with reduced peri-procedural transfusion rate (OR: 0.10; $P < 0.00001$) and reduced duration of post-operative catheterisation following PVP (mean difference: 32.36 h; $P < 0.00001$). Accordingly, the length of stay was shorter relative to the TURP patients (mean difference: 32.36 hours; $P < 0.00001$). Post-procedural re-catheterisation and urinary tract infection rates were comparable in the two groups [11]. Long-term comparative outcome data were not available between the two groups beyond 12 months in these series. Very few prospective studies have addressed this in large prostates over 100 mL.

A prospective multicentre non-randomised study of GreenLIght XPS showed excellent outcomes and safety in a group of over 200 patients of whom the majority were on some form of ongoing anticoagulation and over a quarter had prostate volumes greater than 80 mL [12].

Skolarikos et al. report outcomes of GreenLight laser prostatectomy (n = 65) compared against a control arm of OP (n = 60) for patients with prostate volumes greater than 80 mL in their prospective RCT. 7.7% of the GreenLight laser group required additional intraoperative conversion to TURP for haemostasis. Overall 18-month follow-up results corroborated with earlier data showing a statistically significant shorter period of hospitalisation and catheterisation post-procedure, with non-inferior functional outcomes for GreenLight laser [13].

One concern is the perceived need for 'retreatment' of patients undergoing GreenLight laser prostatectomy. An RCT by Al-Ansari et al. cited re-operation rates of as high as 11% over 36 months; all were in prostate volumes greater than 80 mL [14]. However the energy used in this study was not reported. Interestingly, 3-year outcome data from an American multicentre evaluation of the technique demonstrated a re-intervention rate for Greenlight HPS of 4.3%, however there was no sub-group analysis of the effect of prostate volume on this rate [15].

The meta-analysis by Teng et al. confirmed a higher re-intervention rate than those in the TURP groups studied (RR = 0.24, 95% CI: 0.10–0.59, $P = 0.002$) [10]. It should be noted however, that although bigger glands may display a correlation with a higher rate of retreatment in initial series, the question for future trials (assessing XPS) should address whether adequate energy per mL of prostate tissue was delivered.

The topic of sexual dysfunction in relation to GreenLight laser prostatectomy in large glands over 100 mL is poorly characterised in the literature. As with all surgical modalities for BOO, this is in part related to the co-existence of LUTS and erectile dysfunction. Theoretically, efficacious bladder outflow obstruction surgery relieves LUTS and thus the need to take 5-ARI and/or alpha blockers, which are associated independently with libido reduction and retrograde/anejaculation respectively. The randomised prospective trial by Horasanli et al. (n = 81) demonstrated similar rates of retrograde ejaculation rates in TURP (56.7%) and GreenLight laser groups (49.9% p = 0.21) at 36-months follow-up [16]. In comparison with HoLEP, the rate of retrograde ejaculation in previously sexually active patients within a prospective RCT was significantly lower in GreenLight PVP (28.5% vs. 88%) [17]. The authors felt this reflected the extent of tissue removal in the two groups.

It has been postulated that laser ablation of prostatic tissue, which requires augmented laser energy per unit of prostate, may have a detrimental effect on adjacent cavernous nerves and thus influence sexual function. This is thought to be due to increased transmitted heat which may extend beyond the penetration depth of the laser [18]. Capsular perforation is known to be an independent risk factor for erectile dysfunction in prostatic resection; the extent of penile nerve damage has been established in previous studies evaluating TURP with neurophysiological testing [19].

Elshal et al., in a longitudinal study, propose that post-operative erectile dysfunction is perceived to be more significant in patients with previously normal function prior to GreenLight Laser prostatectomy [18]. This effect has not been confirmed in other multicentre studies which have stringently assessed sexual function. Contemporary erectile dysfunction rates are reported as less than 1% with GreenLight PVP [12, 20] a rate which is reflected in our own clinical practice. We do however support the role of pre-operative sexual function assessment and counselling for all patients.

8.5   Photoselective Vaporization of the Prostate in the Very Large Prostate

There remains distinct heterogeneity in the literature regarding the exact definition of a 'large' prostate. Big glands are associated with a rapid rate of adenomatous enlargement [21, 22]. There is no consensus on exactly how prostate volume should determine surgical approach.

Data specifically examining the use of PVP in the larger prostate is limited. Rajbabu et al. published a contemporary prospective series of 54 patients with BOO whose prostates were greater than 100 mL in size (mean: 135 mL, range 100–300 mL). Their results confirmed that the 80 W KTP laser PVP led to sustained improvements in flow rate. The mean (SD) improvement in Qmax was 8.0 (3.1) to 18.2 (8.1), 18.5 (9.2), 17.9 (7.8) and 19.3 (9.8) mL/s at 3, 6, 12 and 24 months respectively. The IPSS and Quality of life scores demonstrated a similarly favourable trend post-procedure [23]. Despite using only the 80 W laser and despite many of these patients having significant co-morbidities, excellent safety and medium-term results were demonstrated.

At the time of writing, the GOLIATH study is the only published multicentre, multinational RCT to evaluate the XPS 180 W PVP. This was found to be non-inferior to TURP in relation to functional outcomes of IPSS, Qmax and complication rates at 6 months [24]. Subsequent 2-year follow up data [20] confirmed consistent durable effectiveness and safety compared to TURP, irrespective of prostate size. It should be noted however, that men with prostates larger than 100 mL were excluded from this study on the basis of TURP being potentially unsafe for them. GLXPS (n = 136): mean prostate volume: 48.6 mL ± 19.2 mL (SD) versus TURP (n = 133) mean volume: 46.2 ± 19.1 mL (SD). Nonetheless, bleeding related complications and recovery were significantly better in the GreenLight laser group.

Early results from a small (n = 35), single centre series using 180 W GreenLight PVP in prostates greater than 100 mL (median: 132, Range: 118-157 mL) retrospectively reported promising equivalent outcomes to previous trials comparing PVP with the other modalities of TURP and OP at 3 and 6 months. Of note, 31% of this cohort were taking anticoagulants (which were not withheld). There were no blood transfusions required in this series [25].

Araki et al. undertook a prospective evaluation of GreenLight laser in patients on medical therapy for BPH. It has previously been suggested that the downregulation of prostatic angiogenesis in patients on long term 5-alpha reductase inhibitors may affect the efficiency of GreenLight laser usage. This study demonstrated no significant difference in laser time/total energy usage and comparable outcomes in the presence and absence of 5-ARI supplementation [26].

The effectiveness of GreenLight in patients on anticoagulation has generated interest amongst researchers. Sandu et al. undertook a retrospective cohort analysis of 24 men with a mean prostate volume of 82 cc (range 34–164 cc). Each was in receipt of anticoagulation and underwent GreenLight laser PVP. Warfarin was held for 2 days pre-operatively, aspirin and clopidogrel were not stopped in the remaining patients. None of these high-risk cardiac patients had clinically significant hae-maturia, clot retention or thromboembolic events post-operatively. All patients were discharged within 23 h and 92% of men had successful trial without catheter prior to discharge [27].

More recently, the outcome data from GreenLight laser PVP in specific patient groups was published from a larger multi-centre prospective study (n = 305) by Woo et al.; it included anticoagulated patients (n = 62) and those with prostate volumes of >80 mL (n = 52); (mean = 118.4 mL, SD = 34.9 mL). There was a 233.3% improvement in Qmax for patients with prostate volumes greater than 80 mL (mean: 5.8 mL/s SD: 3.4) at baseline compared to follow up at mean follow up of 4.2 months (mean: 19.7 mL/s SD: 9.1). 185% improvement was reported in those with a pros-tate volume of less than 80 mL at baseline (mean: 7.6 mL/s SD 4.4) and at follow up (mean: 21.7 mL/s SD: 10.3).

Clavien-Dindo complications (>2) were comparable in prevalence in both small and larger prostates. There was no statistical difference in functional outcome between those taking versus not taking anticoagulation. There was a 50.8% reduc-tion in prostate volume for those on anticoagulation (mean 72.7 mL SD 36.8 at baseline and 35.8 SD16.2 at follow up), and a 44.2% reduction for those not on anticoagulation (mean: 58.2 SD 33.1 and 32.5 SD 17.4 at baseline and follow up respectively). There was no significant difference in length of stay and period of catheterisation post-procedure between prostate volume groups [28].

Although this study was limited by its mean follow-up time of 4.2 months, it was concluded that unlike TURP, anticoagulation is not a contraindication for GreenLight laser prostatectomy and should be considered routinely in high risk cardiac patients.

In our experience, increasing prostate size correlates with an increase in opera-tive duration and energy utilisation with GreenLight Laser PVP. This has signifi-cantly improved with the introduction of the 180 W XPS laser fibre and will continue to do so with ongoing modifications. We believe that the key technical consideration in managing prostates >100 cc is the creation of the working channel to optimise irrigation flow and thus vision (Fig. 8.3). This can be achieved following early vaporisation of occlusive lateral lobes. If a significant middle lobe is evident, avoid undue pivotal movements at the bladder neck as this can precipitate bleeding and impair the visual field. Sometimes, visualisation of the ureteric orifices must be deferred until the middle lobe has been reduced.

We believe that any surgeon proficient in TURP would find it straightforward to adapt to the GreenLight laser technique, following demonstration of competency in the simulation setting. It is important that the surgeon is patient when commencing GreenLight laser, as the sweep speed required is slower and working distance increased compared to that associated with a loop resectoscope. The mechanics of the technique involve co-ordination of the dominant and non-dominant hands to control the scope and fibre respectively. We recommend from experience that larger glands should not be tackled until fully confident operating on smaller prostates.

The EAU guidelines support GreenLight laser as a "safe method for volume reduction in large sized prostate glands" and "safe and effective for patients receiv-

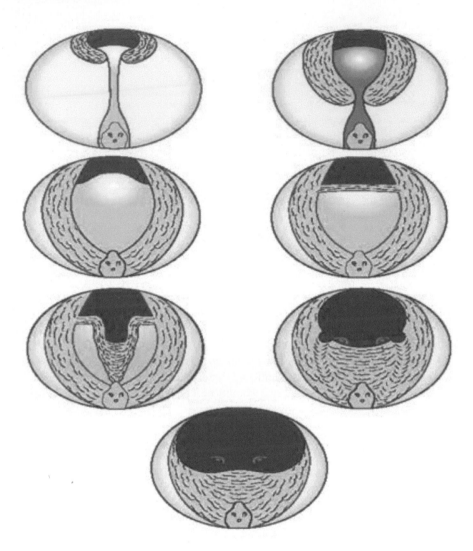

Fig. 8.3 Schematic for creating the working channel with GreenLight laser: An adaptation of the IGLU (International GreenLight Users group) modular technique [4]

ing anticoagulation medication or patients in retention" [29]. In 2016, The National Institute of Health and Clinical Excellence (NICE) issued a resource impact report in which GreenLight XPS was compared with TURP. Cost-modelling analysis estimated a cost-reduction potential of £60 per GreenLight patient. Extrapolating their data on the basis of proportional day case procedures in low-risk patients for both modalities, they predicted an annual saving with PVP of £2.3 million in NHS England [30]. Table 8.1 describes the advantages and disadvantages of GreenLight PVP compared to conventional TURP.

Table 8.1 Advantages of GreenLight PVP versus conventional TURP

Advantages	Disadvantages
True day case operation. Can treat large glands in single procedure	Long term follow up data awaited regarding sustained benefit of PVP
Safe in patients on anticoagulation	MoXy Fibre cannot be used for laser lithotripsy
No risk of TUR syndrome in spite of prolonged vaporisation time in large prostates	TURP skills not directly transferrable. Surgeons need additional simulation training to overcome the learning curve
Catheter free within 24 h	

8.6   Discussion

The 'big prostate' remains a significant benign urological pathology, commonly requiring surgical intervention. The number of patients referred for operative management is likely to increase with an ageing population. Within an elderly population, the proportion of men with significant comorbidities who need surgery is likely to increase. It is not uncommon that patients referred for surgery are on long-term anticoagulation. A modality such as GreenLight Laser, which affords a reduced risk of bleeding that negates the need for bridging therapy and demonstrates comparable functional outcomes in a day case setting is an exciting prospect.

In an ideal world, emerging prospective, well-designed RCTs would directly compare GreenLight laser prostatectomy against all operative modalities for large volume BPH. Funding and cohort heterogeneity make recruitment difficult. Current outcome data available support the efficacious, non-inferiority of laser ablative therapy in the management of large prostates in the long-term. Table 8.2 describes some of the main studies comparing Greenlight PVP with other treatment modalities for the large prostate.

As with the adoption of any new surgical technique, the use of simulation in the context of a formal, certified training programme with synchronous mentorship, is recommended to improve the procedure-specific aptitude, safety profile and confidence of the surgeon undertaking GreenLight laser prostatectomy in large prostates.

It could be argued that patients with very large prostates should only be managed in centres where a number of the modern management techniques for large prostates are offered. We believe that a bespoke approach respecting each patient's status and aspirations will allow the best outcomes in this difficult group of patients.

8.7   Conclusion

GreenLight laser is a very safe option even for men with significant co-morbidities and can be offered to almost any man with LUTS or retention regardless of prostate size or general health status. In both of our centres it is routine to manage high risk and anticoagulated patients with prostates over 100 mL as outpatient day case

Table 8.2 Comparative GreenLight PVP studies in large prostates/high risk patients

Trial	Number of patients and trial design	Main inclusion/ exclusion criteria	Intervention(s)	Relevant outcomes
Bachmann et al., Thomas et al. (GOLIATH trial) 2014 and 2016 [20, 24]	n = 281 Multicentre Randomised, non-inferiority comparative trial	Prostates >100 cc excluded from trial	GreenLight XPS 180 W PVP or TURP	GLXPS non-inferior to TURP for IPSS, Qmax and complication rate at 6 and 24 month follow up
Woo et al. 2008 [28]	n = 305 Multicentre prospective study	Subgroup analysis: 63 patients in urinary retention, 70 patients on anticoagulation, 52 patients with prostate volume > 80 cc	GreenLight HPS 120 W	GLHPS is Safe and efficacious in patients on anticoagulation with comparable short term complication rates
Skolarikos et al. 2008 [13]	n = 125 Randomised prospective study	Prostates >80 cc included	GreenLight PVP or Open Prostatectomy (OP)	Shorter hospital stay, length of catheterization, perioperative blood loss and equivocal short term functional outcomes in GLPVP vs. OP
Rajbabu et al. 2007 [23]	n = 53 Single centre prospective study	Prostates >100 cc (mean 135, range 100–300) included	GreenLight KTP 80 W	Mean catheterization time 23 h (0–72 h) Sustained favourable IPSS and Qmax at 2 year follow up

procedures, often sending even these patients home without a catheter. Risks of bleeding, perforation and incontinence are very small. The early benefits need to be set against what will likely be a longer-term re-operation rate that is higher than for full laser enucleation. However for those more elderly men the rates of reoperation at 10–20 years may not be as important.

References

1. Kuntzman RS, Malek RS, Barrett DM, Bostwick DG. Potassium-titanyl-phosphate laser vaporization of the prostate: a comparative functional and pathologic study in canines. Urology. 1996;48(4):575–83.
2. Bachmann A, Ruszat R. The KTP-(greenlight-) laser—principles and experiences. Minim Invasive Ther Allied Technol. 2007;16(1):5–10.

3. Malek RS, Barrett DM, Kuntzman RS. High-power potassium-titanyl-phosphate (KTP/532) laser vaporization prostatectomy: 24 hours later. Urology. 1998;51(2):254–6.
4. Muir G, Gómez Sancha F, Bachmann A, Choi B, Collins E, de la Rosette J, et al. Techniques and Training with GreenLight HPS 120-W Laser Therapy of the Prostate: Position Paper. Eur Urol Suppl. 2008;7(4):370–7.
5. Ben-Zvi T, Hueber PA, Liberman D, Valdivieso R, Zorn KC. GreenLight XPS 180W vs HPS 120W laser therapy for benign prostate hyperplasia: a prospective comparative analysis after 200 cases in a single-center study. Urology. 2013;81(4):853–8.
6. Heinrich E, Schiefelbein F, Schoen G. Technique and Short-Term Outcome of Green Light Laser (KTP, 80 W) Vaporisation of the Prostate. Eur Urol. 2007;52(6):1632–7.
7. Hueber P-A, Liberman D, Ben-Zvi T, Woo H, Hai MA, Te AE, et al. 180 W vs 120 W Lithium triborate photoselective vaporization of the prostate for benign prostatic hyperplasia: a global, multicenter comparative analysis of perioperative treatment parameters. Urology. 2013;82(5):1108–13.
8. Barber NJ, Zhu G, Donohue JF, Thompson PM, Walsh K, Muir GH. Use of expired breath ethanol measurements in evaluation of irrigant absorption during high-power potassium titanyl phosphate laser vaporization of prostate. Urology. 2006;67(1):80–3.
9. Seki N, Nomura H, Yamaguchi A, Naito S. Evaluation of the learning curve for photoselective vaporization of the prostate over the course of 74 cases. J Endourol. 2008;22(8):1731–6.
10. Teng J, Zhang D, Li Y, Yin L, Wang K, Cui X, et al. Photoselective vaporization with the green light laser vs transurethral resection of the prostate for treating benign prostate hyperplasia: a systematic review and meta-analysis. BJU Int. 2013;111(2):312–23.
11. Cornu J-N, Ahyai S, Bachmann A, de la Rosette J, Gilling P, Gratzke C, et al. A Systematic review and meta-analysis of functional outcomes and complications following transurethral procedures for lower urinary tract symptoms resulting from benign prostatic obstruction: an update. Eur Urol. 2015;67(6):1066–96.
12. Bachmann A, Muir GH, Collins EJ, Choi BB, Tabatabaei S, Reich OM, et al. 180-W XPS GreenLight laser therapy for benign prostate hyperplasia: early safety, efficacy, and perioperative outcome after 201 procedures. Eur Urol. 2012;61(3):600–7.
13. Skolarikos A, Papachristou C, Athanasiadis G, Chalikopoulos D, Deliveliotis C, Alivizatos G. Eighteen-month results of a randomized prospective study comparing transurethral photoselective vaporization with transvesical open enucleation for prostatic adenomas greater than 80 cc. J Endourol. 2008;22(10):2333–40.
14. Al-Ansari A, Younes N, Sampige VP, Al-Rumaihi K, Ghafouri A, Gul T, et al. GreenLight HPS 120-W Laser vaporization versus transurethral resection of the prostate for treatment of benign prostatic hyperplasia: a randomized clinical trial with midterm follow-up. Eur Urol. 2010;58(3):349–55.
15. Te AE, Malloy TR, Stein BS, Ulchaker JC, Nseyo UO, Hai MA. Impact of prostate-specific antigen level and prostate volume as predictors of efficacy in photoselective vaporization prostatectomy: analysis and results of an ongoing prospective multicentre study at 3 years. BJU Int. 2006;97(6):1229–33.
16. Horasanli K, Silay MS, Altay B, Tanriverdi O, Sarica K, Miroglu C. Photoselective potassium titanyl phosphate (KTP) laser vaporization versus transurethral resection of the prostate for prostates larger than 70 mL: a short-term prospective randomized trial. Urology. 2008;71(2):247–51.
17. Elmansy H, Baazeem A, Kotb A, Badawy H, Riad E, Emran A, et al. holmium laser enucleation versus photoselective vaporization for prostatic adenoma greater than 60 Ml: preliminary results of a prospective, randomized clinical trial. J Urol. 2012;188(1):216–21.
18. Elshal AM, Elmansy HM, Elkoushy MA, Elhilali MM. Male sexual function outcome after three laser prostate surgical techniques: a single center perspective. Urology. 2012;80(5):1098–104.
19. Lefaucheur JP, Yiou R, Salomon L, Chopin DK, Abbou CC. Assessment of penile small nerve fiber damage after transurethral resection of the prostate by measurement of penile thermal sensation. J Urol. 2000;164(4):1416–9.

20. Thomas JA, Tubaro A, Barber N, d'Ancona F, Muir G, Witzsch U, et al. A multicenter randomized noninferiority trial comparing GreenLight-XPS laser vaporization of the prostate and transurethral resection of the prostate for the treatment of benign prostatic obstruction: Two-yr outcomes of the GOLIATH study. Eur Urol. 2016;69(1):94–102.

21. Lieber MM, Rhodes T, Jacobson DJ, McGree ME, Girman CJ, Jacobsen SJ, et al. Natural history of benign prostatic enlargement: long-term longitudinal population-based study of prostate volume doubling times. BJU Int. 2010;105(2):214–9.

22. Rhodes T, Girman CJ, Jacobsen SJ, Roberts RO, Guess HA, Lieber MM. Longitudinal prostate growth rates during 5 years in randomly selected community men 40 to 79 years old. J Urol. 1999;161(4):1174–9.

23. Rajbabu K, Chandrasekara SK, Barber NJ, Walsh K, Muir GH. Photoselective vaporization of the prostate with the potassium-titanyl-phosphate laser in men with prostates of >100 mL. BJU Int. 2007;100(3):593–8; discussion 8.

24. Bachmann A, Tubaro A, Barber N, d'Ancona F, Muir G, Witzsch U, et al. 180-W XPS GreenLight laser vaporisation versus transurethral resection of the prostate for the treatment of benign prostatic obstruction: 6-month safety and efficacy results of a European Multicentre Randomised trial—the GOLIATH study. Eur Urol. 2014;65(5):931–42.

25. Nicholson H, Woo H. The massively enlarged prostate: experience with photoselective vaporization of the ≥100 cc prostate using the 180 W lithium triborate laser. J Endourol. 2014;29(4):459–62.

26. Araki M, Lam PN, Culkin DJ, Wong C. Decreased efficiency of potassium-titanyl-phosphate laser photoselective vaporization prostatectomy with long-term 5 alpha-reductase inhibition therapy: is it true? Urology. 2007;70(5):927–30.

27. Sandhu JS, Ng CK, Gonzalez RR, Kaplan SA, Te AE. Photoselective laser vaporization prostatectomy in men receiving anticoagulants. J Endourol. 2005;19(10):1196–8.

28. Woo H, Reich O, Bachmann A, Choi B, Collins E, de la Rosette J, et al. Outcome of GreenLight HPS 120-W laser therapy in specific patient populations: those in retention, on anticoagulants, and with large prostates (≥80 ml). Eur Urol Suppl. 2008;7(4):378–83.

29. Herrmann TRW, Liatsikos EN, Nagele U, Traxer O, Merseburger AS. EAU Guidelines on Laser Technologies. Eur Urol. 2012;61(4):783–95.

30. NICE. GreenLight XPS for treating benign prostatic hyperplasia: National Institute of Health and Clinical Excellence; 2016. https://www.nice.org.uk/guidance/mtg29/chapter/1-Recommendations.

Chapter 9
Surgical Treatment: Transurethral Resection of the Prostate

Maria Vedanayagam and Ian Dickinson

9.1 Introduction

Transurethral resection of the prostate (TURP) was introduced in the early twentieth century and has since evolved with various adaptations to the technique.

TURP is currently the standard recommended surgical procedure for men with bothersome lower urinary tract symptoms (LUTS) with prostate sizes between 30 and 80 mL [1]. For prostates larger than 80 mL, retropubic or suprapubic prostatectomy has traditionally been regarded the surgical standard, especially in developing countries [1].

The European Association of Urology (EAU) also recommends Holmium Laser Enucleation of the Prostate (HoLEP) and bipolar enucleation as the current standard for prostates >80 mL. TURP still has a role in this group of patients, although it is not recommended as a first choice by the EAU [1]. This choice is ultimately a result of a discussion between the surgeon and the patient and availability or lack of other treatment modalities. The maximum size of prostate that can be treated by TURP is not defined in the literature. In UK current practice, a TURP can be performed for prostates >100 mL, depending on surgeon experience. The final decision must be made by the operating surgeon at the time of surgery.

The aim of this chapter is to discuss the option of performing a TURP in patients with a large prostate >100 mL, to review the current evidence behind the equipment used, the clinical efficacy and safety of the procedure, and to describe our own approach of using TURP in such cases.

For the purposes of this chapter we have assumed that millilitre (mL), cubic centimeter (cc) and grams (g) are interchangeable.

M. Vedanayagam (✉) • I. Dickinson
Darent Valley Hospital, Darenth Wood Road, Dartford, Kent DA2 8DA, UK
e-mail: Maria.vedanayagam@nhs.net; ikdickinson@mac.com

© Springer International Publishing AG 2018   117
V. Kasivisvanathan, B. Challacombe (eds.), *The Big Prostate*,
https://doi.org/10.1007/978-3-319-64704-3_9

9.2   Choice of TURP Over Other Treatments for the Very Large Prostate Greater Than 100 cc

Open prostatectomy (OP) was traditionally performed for the management of the large prostate causing benign prostatic obstruction. In the advent of minimally invasive surgery, HoLEP is now recommended [1]. A randomized controlled trial (RCT) of HoLEP versus OP in >100 g prostates demonstrated that HoLEP was a suitable minimally invasive alternative [2]. Comparatively, HoLEP had shorter hospital stays, shorter catheterization time and similar postoperative outcomes to OP, but a significantly longer operating time [3–5].

When comparing open prostatectomy and TURP, in experienced hands, a surgeon may have a personal preference for a TURP from an operative point of view but also may favour this option because of a shorter hospital stay and reduced costs associated with TURP. Patients will also usually prefer a minimally invasive option associated with a shorter recovery period and hospital stay [6, 7]. An increase in morbidity and mortality has been shown with a resection weight of >60 g following a TURP [8].

A study comparing the post-operative outcomes of bipolar TURP (B-TURP) and suprapubic open prostatectomy (SP) on prostates over 100 g in patients >65 years showed that mean catheter time and hospital stay was significant less in the B-TURP group, however operative time was significantly more (102.8 min versus 73.5 min) [7]. Clinical efficacy assessed by IPSS, quality of life (QoL), peak-flow rate, postvoid residual (PVR), and International Index of Erectile Function (IIEF-5) scores at 12 months showed no statistically significant difference, supporting the use of B-TURP for 100 g prostates [7]. In certain cases, the surgeon may be unable to complete the procedure in one sitting either due to poor visibility or prolonged resection time. Prolonged resection times increases the risk of fluid absorption, subsequent dilutional hyponatraemia and particularly in the case of monopolar TURP (M-TURP) using glycine, increases the risk of TUR(P) syndrome which is a urological emergency, Patients should therefore be counselled about the possibility of a two stage procedure should the surgeon encounter such difficulties [9].

One of the major advantages of TURP is that access to the equipment and availability of training in the technique is greater than some of the other endoscopic techniques used to manage the big prostate. From a health-service delivery point of view, it is one of the more feasible options available for management the big prostate. Despite this there are some limitations of the technique. In large prostates, a RCT demonstrated that HoLEP removed greater volumes of tissue (40 g vs. 24.7 g), had shorter catheterisation times and hospital stay in comparison to TURP. The operative time however was longer and no significant difference was observed in improvement of the maximum flow rate (Q_{max}) and International Prostate Symptom Score (IPSS) [10]. Unlike with TURP, a large case series showed that the outcomes of HoLEP were independent of size [11]. An additional benefit of HoLEP to consider in the large prostate, is that it can be performed in patients on anti-coagulation or antiplatelet medication [12]. According to the NICE guidelines, HoLEP can be offered to patients in a centre that specialises in the technique or in one with a mentorship programme in place [13]. This limits its availability.

Photoselective vaporization of the prostate (PVP) using the GreenLight® system can also be used to surgically manage the >100 mL prostate. A small study assessing the efficacy of PVP on large prostates (mean 135 g) showed an improvement in IPSS and QoL with a 7% rate of post-operative clot retention [14]. A systematic review, irrespective of prostate size, showed that PVP had similar efficacy to TURP with reduced rates of blood transfusion, catheterisation time and hospital stay [15]. A small study comparing TURP and PVP in large prostates between 70–100 mL favoured PVP in terms of a shorter catheterisation time and hospital stay. An 8% transfusion rate was seen in the TURP group compared to 0% in the PVP group. In terms of efficacy, a significant improvement in IPSS and Q_{max}, favouring TURP was demonstrated, however this study was limited by a short follow-up period of 6 months [16]. Equal clinical efficacy was demonstrated in a longer follow up study of 24 months [17]. PVP can be used safely in patients on anti-coagulation, unlike for TURP, and in those with a large prostate >80 cc [18].

In summary, of the techniques discussed, we recommend choosing the surgical procedure the surgeon is most comfortable performing when tackling the >100 mL prostate. Surgeons should take into consideration the availability of equipment, cost of the procedure, length of patient stay, ease of training and patient wishes. For patients on anticoagulation that cannot be stopped, PVP or HoLEP can be considered. In grossly enlarged glands, estimated at >150 cc, we recommend HoLEP or open prostatectomy as an alternative. We prefer to use TURP over PVP as we feel better haemostatic control with large glands has been observed. In centres where HoLEP is not available, or the patient has multiple co-morbidities where prolonged surgical time is a concern, a less invasive TURP or hemi-TURP may prove the best option.

For a summary of trials comparing the outcomes of TURP for large prostates compared to other treatment modalities please see Table 9.1.

Table 9.1 A table showing trials comparing the outcomes of TURP for large prostates compared to other treatment modalities

Trial	Number of patients and trial design	Interventions	Mean prostate weight	Statistically significant outcomes
Coskuner et al. (2014) [7]	Retrospective study N = 102	B-TURP vs. Open SP	120 mL vs. 116 mL	– Shorter post-operative catheterisation time – Shorter hospital stay – Longer operative time – No difference in clinical efficacy

(continued)

Table 9.1 (continued)

Trial	Number of patients and trial design	Interventions	Mean prostate weight	Statistically significant outcomes
Giulianelli et al. (2011) [6]	Randomised trial	B-TURP vs. Open SP	83.3 mL vs. 84.3 mL	– Shorter post-operative catheterisation time – Shorter hospital stay – No difference in clinical efficacy
Tan et al. (2003) [10]	RCT N = 61	TURP vs. HoLEP	70 mL (46–152) vs. 77 mL (42–152)	– Longer post-operative catheterisation time – Longer hospital stay – Shorter operative time – Equal clinical efficacy at 12 months
Tasci et al. (2008) [17]	Non-randomised bicenter trial N = 81	TURP vs. PVP	104.2 mL vs. 108.4 mL	– Longer post-operative catheterisation time – Shorter operative time – Longer hospital stay – No difference in clinical efficacy at 24 months
Horasanil et al. (2008) [16]	Randomized trial N = 76	TURP vs. PVP	88 mL vs. 86 mL	– Longer post-operative catheterisation time – Shorter operative time – Longer hospital stay – Improved clinical efficacy at 6 months – Lower re-intervention rate at 6 months – Higher rate of blood transfusion

Table 9.1 (continued)

Kuntz et al. (2002, 2008) [2, 3]	RCT N = 120	HoLE P vs. Open SP	114.6 mL vs. 113 mL	– Shorter post-operative catheterisation time – Shorter hospital stay – Longer operative time – Less blood loss – No difference in clinical efficacy

B-TURP bipolar TURP, *SP* suprapubic prostatectomy, *RCT* randomised controlled trial, *HoLEP* holmium laser enucleation of the prostate, *PVP* photoselective vaporisation of the prostate, *Open SP* open simple prostatectomy
Clinical efficacy refers to IPPS, Q_{max} and PVR

9.3   Evaluating Prostate Size

The prostate size is initially evaluated by digital rectal examination (DRE), however as the prostate enlarges, particularly >30 cc, DRE alone can underestimate the true size [19]. Prior to planning surgical treatment, the EAU recommends imaging by transrectal ultrasound (TRUS) or transabdominal ultrasound to estimate prostate size. A study showed that transabdominal ultrasound overestimated the prostate size by 55.7% while TRUS slightly underestimated the weight by 4.4% [20]. This has also been reflected in the experience of the author where prostate sizes estimated at >100 cc on transabdominal ultrasound have been smaller on cystoscopic inspection. In such cases where the prostate size has been estimated as very large, a TRUS, or if available, a multi parametric MRI, may be a better option to accurately plan for surgery.

9.4   Equipment

Using a continuous flow resectoscope, monopolar TURP (M-TURP) relies on electrical current flowing in one direction to cut the tissue with a wire loop. A grounding pad must be attached to the patient (the return electrode) and a clear, non-conducting inert fluid; commonly 1.5% glycine is used. Glycine however is hypo-osmolar and can cause dilutional hyponatraemia and TUR syndrome if there is systemic absorption of the irrigant, especially seen with capsular perforation. Surgical resection time is usually limited to 60 min to reduce the risk of such complications. This may thus reduce the amount that can be resected therefore limiting the size of prostate that can be treated by M-TURP.

Bipolar TURP (B-TURP) uses isotonic saline for irrigation and subsequently is associated with a lower risk of TUR syndrome. It is also thought to have better hae-mostatic abilities as some studies have suggested that a deeper coagulative effect is achieved with bipolar energy [21]. This may allow a more prolonged resection time and hence augment the ability to resect larger prostates >100 mL.

There are different systems available, all of which rely on the active electrode on the cutting loop wire which transmits energy to the sodium ions of the irrigating fluid to form a plasma corona vaporisation field which cleaves the tissue to allow resection [22, 23]. The point at which they differ is the location of the return electrode; In the Plasma Kinetic (PK) system (Gyrus ACMI) this is on the loop itself, and there-fore a lower voltage is required to generate a current. In the TURis system (Olympus), the return electrode is on the inner sheath of the resectoscope itself. The diameter of the cutting wire loop in B-TURP sets is smaller than that used for M-TURP.

There have been several studies comparing the safety and efficacy of M-TURP versus B-TURP. A meta-analysis of randomised controlled trials (RCT) comparing B-TURP with M-TURP showed no significant difference in the clinical effective-ness seen in post-operative IPSS and Q_{max} [24]. M-TURP had increased adverse events of TURP syndrome, none were reported in the B-TURP group. A higher frequency of clot retention was also reported in the M-TURP group, a finding reflected in previous systematic reviews [24, 25].

In 2012, an international multicentre double-blind randomized controlled trial considering the safety and efficacy of B-TURP versus M-TURP showed no clinical advantage of B-TURP. In terms of adverse events, a decrease in post-operative sodium levels was seen following M-TURP. This may suggest that especially in training cases, B-TURP may be safer in inexperienced/training hands as it theoreti-cally allows an increased time for resection and subsequently would be preferable when tackling the 100 mL prostate when is it is difficult to restrict surgical time to 60 min [26, 27]. A Post Hoc analysis of this study for patients with large prostates, showed that for a mean prostate volume of approximately 108 mL, the rates for safety and clinical efficacy remained comparable in M-TURP and B-TURP. The drop in post-operative sodium seen with M-TURP remained a significant difference but was not clinically translated into a significant difference in TUR syndrome [28].

The issue of post-operative urethral strictures remains debatable. Komura et al. showed that patients with a large prostate (>70 mL in this study), sustained a significantly higher rate of urethral stricture with B-TURP (TURis in this study) compared to monopolar TURP, this was not seen in the <70 mL prostate sub-group. Interestingly, the strictures that did occur post M-TURP were at the blad-der neck in comparison to the anterior urethra seen with B-TURP [29]. Despite concerns of urethral stricture, clear conclusion cannot be drawn from this study, however it must be acknowledged that unlike the PK system by GYRUS, the TURis is not a true Bipolar system (quasi bipolar system) as the output and collection electrode are not on the wire loop [29]. It has been postulated that perhaps the anterior urethral strictures may be associated with current leak as it travels through the inner sheath [23, 29]. These results were in contrast to the study by Mamoulakis et al. which demonstrated no significant difference between the rates of urethral strictures and bladder neck contractures using the AUTOCON® II 400 ESU system (Karl Storz system), equipped for both bipolar and monopolar output [26, 27].

9.5 Taking on the 100 mL Prostate

When faced with the resection of a 100 cc prostate, preparation is key. The patient should be positioned in the trendelenberg position, level with the edge of the table. We prefer the use of B-TURP with normal saline delivered through an in-line fluid warmer to maintain constant temperature of fluid circulating through the resectosope. This maintains a constant core temperature of the patient and optimises performance of the B-TURP. The fluid height should be kept as low as possible to reduce fluid absorption and preferably no higher than 60 cm above the level of the pubic symphysis. This is more important when using M-TURP with hypo-osmolar irrigating fluid. Surgeon comfort should be optimised with preferably a foot operated pneumatic mobile stool and the screen centred over the patient's head.

Pre-operative imaging with ultrasound or MRI is advised to plan surgery. Prior to surgery, start with digital rectal examination to gauge the size of the prostate. A diagnostic cystoscopy should be performed to assess urethral calibre, location of the verumontanum, a pivotal landmark for the procedure, size and vascularity of the prostate, taking care not to cause bleeding before starting the procedure. In the case of the very large prostate, the apical lobes may extend below the level of the verumontanum and it is important here to identify the distal limit of resection as the cystoscope is advanced. On entry into the bladder, look out for a large middle lobe or intravesical extension of the prostate which may obscure the vision of the ureteric orifices. The bladder walls should also be visualised to rule out other pathology.

A 26Ch resectoscope using a visual obturator should be inserted. Care is taken to distend the bladder away from any large intravesical prostatic lobes prior to resection. Different techniques have been described which mainly differ in the order in which the adenomatous tissue is resected. When attempting such large prostates, the surgeon should always choose a technique they are familiar with, that is sequential. We describe our preferred method for the purposes of this chapter.

Start with the middle lobe working from one side of the lobe to the other in the same line until the ring of muscle fibres at the bladder neck is clearly defined—this is the proximal limit. Once this is achieved, all resections should be distal to this. Resection beyond this may undermine the trigone or result in resection of the ureteric orifices. It is imperative in cases of a prominent middle lobe to re-evaluate the location of the ureteric orifices intermittently.

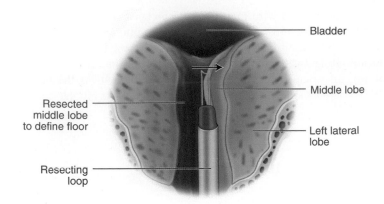

Fig. 9.1 This illustrates the start of the procedure commenced by working across one side of the middle lobe to the other

We recommend working across one side of the middle lobe to the other, each time progressing distally towards the apex until the verumontanum is reached—this is the distal limit. This technique leaves the operator with a smooth floor without prominent irregularities of adenomatous tissue (Fig. 9.1) and improves flow through the resectoscope thus improving vision.

Once the floor of the prostate has been resected, move on to the left lateral lobe. This should be divided into lower half and upper half. Starting at 5 o'clock, moving anticlockwise towards the 3 o'clock position and then back down to the starting point until the same level as the floor (resected middle lobe) is reached (Fig. 9.2). This is repeated, moving distally until the apex is reached. Sometimes, the lateral lobes are seen to protrude below the level of the verumontanum and can distort the sphincter. Having resected the upper half of the lobe, proceed to the lower half starting at 3 o'clock and resecting round to 6 o'clock resect back to the level of the verumontanum.

During each resection, try to achieve canoe-shaped chips as described by Blandy [30]. That is, chips as wide as they are deep and their length determined by the length travelled by the loop. This can be increased by carefully moving the resectoscope back in large prostates ensuring the surgeon is always aware of the location of the external urethral sphincter [30]. Note that the chips produced by B-TURP are smaller due to vaporisation and a smaller sized loop.

Throughout the procedure, keep track of time, if you find, that it has taken over 45 min to resect one lobe, a hemi-resection may be in the best interest of the patient. The role of hemi-TURP has been described as resection of one lateral lobe and median lobe, if present. This creates a clear channel and can be used as a means of reducing operative time and bleeding in the high risk patient [23]. This systematic approach yields better outcomes if the surgeon has to terminate the operation early due to poor vision from increased bleeding, or fluid

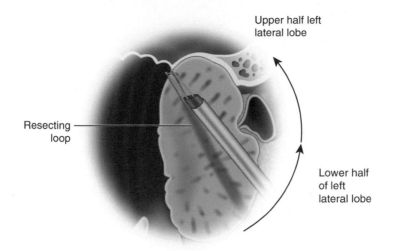

Fig. 9.2 This illustrates how the lateral lobes should be tackled if starting on the left-hand side of the prostate; starting at 5 o'clock, moving anticlockwise towards the 3 o'clock position to reach the same level as the floor of the resected middle lobes

absorption if they are only able to completely resect one lobe. Focus on removing the bulk of the obstructing tissue and avoid the temptation of random resection of other parts of the prostate. A single centre, prospective, randomized study comparing outcomes of TURP and open surgery for prostate volumes over 80 mL showed that in 42% of cases, TURP procedure had to be completed in two sessions, even in experienced hands secondary to poor vision or prolonged resection time [9].

Hemi-resection performed in prostates >120 g achieved patient satisfaction in terms of lower urinary tract symptom improvement but was associated with a higher UTI and re-admission rate [31]. Resection of <30% of prostatic tissue versus >50% still achieved a significant improvement in IPSS and QoL [32]. In the high-risk patient troubled by LUTS, who does not want or is not suitable for a long-term catheter, a hemi-TURP can be planned to improve IPSS or achieve catheter free voiding, in those who a prolonged or second anaesthetic is unfavourable. In cases where a hemi-resection was performed due to prolonged surgical time or poor vision, a completion TURP should be performed at the surgeons and anaesthetist's discretion.

Once the left lateral lobe is completed, use the same technique for the right lateral lobe moving clockwise and anticlockwise migrating distally from the bladder neck to the apex to reach the same level of resection. To complete the resection, move the scope to just below the level of the verumontanum and look up to the bladder, any remaining obstructing tissue should be removed and can be achieved by holding the resectoscope stationary at this point to avoid injury to the sphincter (Fig. 9.3).

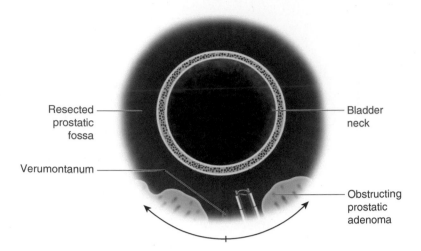

Fig. 9.3 This illustrates the view one should aim to achieve when looking from the verumontanum towards the bladder neck, where protruding adenoma can be resected to achieve a clear channel

When the resected prostatic chips fall into the prostatic fossa obscuring view, an Ellik evacuator should be used to remove the chips. This interruption to the rhythm needed when resecting large prostates should be kept to a minimum. The author prefers the use of a disposable Ellik with a flap valve, which prevents evacuated tissue from re-entering the bladder.

Meticulous haemostasis in the case of the 100 mL prostate is paramount. Communicate with the anaesthetist to ensure the blood pressure (BP) is not significantly lower than the pre-operative BP. Reducing the in-flow fluid allows one to identify any remaining bleeding vessels. This can be achieved with the loop, button or roller-ball depending on surgeon preference and availability.

The procedure should be complete with the insertion of an indwelling 22 Fr 3-way catheter with 50 mL in the balloon to prevent its migration into the prostatic cavity and continuous irrigation with 0.9% saline should be used. All patients should have a post-operative blood test to include full blood count and serum electrolytes.

Careful instructions should be given to the recovery nurse and highlighted on the operative notes regarding the need for continuous irrigation to be maintained, if necessary, overnight. If there are concerns of bleeding, initially catheter traction and manual bladder washouts may be necessary.

9.6   Conclusion

The choice of surgical management of the >100 mL prostate ultimately lies with surgeon experience and must be made after a careful assessment of the patient's co-morbidities, estimated prostate size and patient concerns and wishes. In experienced hands a TURP can be performed safely and effectively. In grossly enlarged glands >150 mL, we recommend open prostatectomy or HoLEP.

References

1. S. Gravas, T. Bach, A. Bachmann, M. Drake, M. Gacci, C. Gratzke, S. Madersbacher, C. Mamoulakis. K.A.O.T.EAU guidelines on non-neurogenic male LUTS including benign prostatic obstruction. 2016. https://uroweb.org/guideline/treatment-of-non-neurogenic-male-luts/?type=pocket-guidelines

2. Kuntz RM, Lehrich K, Ahyai SA. Holmium laser enucleation of the prostate versus open prostatectomy for prostates greater than 100 grams: 5-year follow-up results of a randomised clinical trial. Eur Urol. 2008;53:160–8.

3. Kuntz RM, Lehrich K. Transurethral holmium laser enucleation versus transvesical open enucleation for prostate adenoma greater than 100 gm: a randomized prospective trial of 120 patients. J Urol. 2002;168:1465–9.

4. Lin Y, et al. Transurethral enucleation of the prostate versus transvesical open prostatectomy for large benign prostatic hyperplasia: a systematic review and meta-analysis of randomized controlled trials. World J Urol. 2016;34:1207–19.

5. Li M, et al. Endoscopic enucleation versus open prostatectomy for treating large benign prostatic hyperplasia: a meta-analysis of randomized controlled trials. PLoS One. 2015;10:e0121265.

6. Giulianelli R, et al. Comparative randomized study on the efficaciousness of treatment of BOO due to BPH in patients with prostate up to 100 gr by endoscopic gyrus prostate resection versus open prostatectomy. Preliminary data. Arch Ital Urol Androl. 2011;83:88–94.

7. Coskuner ER, Ozkan TA, Koprulu S, Dillioglugil O, Cevik I. The role of the bipolar plasmakinetic TURP over 100 g prostate in the elderly patients. Int Urol Nephrol. 2014;46:2071–7.

8. Reich O, et al. Morbidity, mortality and early outcome of transurethral resection of the prostate: a prospective multicenter evaluation of 10,654 patients. J Urol. 2008;180:246–9.

9. Persu C, et al. TURP for BPH. How large is too large? J Med Life. 2010;3:376–80.

10. Tan AH, et al. A randomized trial comparing holmium laser enucleation of the prostate with transurethral resection of the prostate for the treatment of bladder outlet obstruction secondary to benign prostatic hyperplasia in large glands (40 to 200 grams). J Urol. 2003;170:1270–4.

11. Elzayat EA, Habib EI, Elhilali MM. Holmium laser enucleation of the prostate: a size-independent new 'gold standard'. Urology. 2005;66:108–13.

12. Herrmann TRW, et al. EAU guidelines on laser technologies. Eur Urol. 2012;61:783–95.

13. Holmium laser prostatectomy | 4-Other-NICE-recommendations-on-holmium-laser-prostatectomy | Guidance and guidelines | NICE. https://www.nice.org.uk/guidance/ipg17/chapter/4-Other-NICE-recommendations-on-holmium-laser-prostatectomy

14. Rajbabu K, Chandrasekara SK, Barber NJ, Walsh K, Muir GH. Photoselective vaporization of the prostate with the potassium-titanyl-phosphate laser in men with prostates of >100 mL. BJU Int. 2007;100:593–8.

15. Teng J, et al. Photoselective vaporization with the green light laser vs transurethral resection of the prostate for treating benign prostate hyperplasia: a systematic review and meta-analysis. BJU Int. 2013;111:312–23.

16. Horasanli K, et al. Photoselective potassium titanyl phosphate (KTP) laser vaporization versus transurethral resection of the prostate for prostates larger than 70 ml: a short-term prospective randomized trial. Urology. 2008;71:247–51.

17. Woo H, et al. Outcome of GreenLight HPS 120-W laser therapy in specific patient populations: those in retention, on anticoagulants, and with large prostates (≥ 80ml). Eur Urol Suppl. 2008;7:378–83.

18. Roehrborn CG. Accurate determination of prostate size via digital rectal examination and transrectal ultrasound. Urology. 1998;51:19–22.

19. Stravodimos KG, et al. TRUS versus transabdominal ultrasound as a predictor of enucleated adenoma weight in patients with BPH: a tool for standard preoperative work-up? Int Urol Nephrol. 2009;41:767–71.

20. Qu L, Wang X, Huang X, Zhang Y, Zeng X. The hemostatic properties of transurethral plasmakinetic resection of the prostate: comparison with conventional resectoscope in an ex vivo study. Urol Int. 2008;80:292–5.

21. S. Gravas, T. Bach, A. Bachmann, M. Drake, M. Gacci, C. Gratzke, S. Madersbacher, C. Mamoulakis, K. A. O. T. EAU guidelines for treatment of non-neurogenic male lower urinary tract symptoms. 2016. https://uroweb.org/guideline/treatment-of-non-neurogenic-male-luts/
22. Smith AD, editor. Smith's textbook of endourology, vol. 1. Oxford: Wiley-Blackwell; 2012.
23. Omar MI, et al. Systematic review and meta-analysis of the clinical effectiveness of bipolar compared with monopolar transurethral resection of the prostate (TURP). BJU Int. 2014;113:24–35.
24. Mamoulakis C, Ubbink DT, de la Rosette JJ. Bipolar versus monopolar transurethral resection of the prostate: a systematic review and meta-analysis of randomized controlled trials. Eur Urol. 2009;56:798–809.
25. Mamoulakis C, et al. Results from an international multicentre double-blind randomized controlled trial on the perioperative efficacy and safety of bipolar vs monopolar transurethral resection of the prostate. BJU Int. 2012;109:240–8.
26. Mamoulakis C, et al. Midterm results from an international multicentre randomised controlled trial comparing bipolar with monopolar transurethral resection of the prostate. Eur Urol. 2013;63:667–76.
27. Skolarikos A, et al. Safety and efficacy of bipolar versus monopolar transurethral resection of the prostate in patients with large prostates or severe lower urinary tract symptoms: post hoc analysis of a european multicenter randomized controlled trial. J Urol. 2016;195:677–84.
28. Komura K, et al. Incidence of urethral stricture after bipolar transurethral resection of the prostate using TURis: Results from a randomised trial. BJU Int. 2015;115:644–52.
29. Blandy JP, Notley RG, Reynard J. Transurethral resection. London: Taylor & Francis; 2005.
30. Abidi SS, Feroz I, Aslam M, Fawad A. Elective hemi transurethral resection of prostate: a safe and effective method of treating huge benign prostatic hyperplasia. J Coll Physicians Surg Pak. 2012;22:35–40.
31. Antunes AA, Srougi M, Coelho RF, Leite KR, Freire Gde C. Transurethral resection of the prostate for the treatment of lower urinary tract symptoms related to benign prostatic hyperplasia: how much should be resected? Int. Braz J Urol 35, 683–9; discussion 689–91.
32. Tasci AI, Tugcu V, Sahin S, Zorluoglu F. Rapid communication: photoselective vaporization of the prostate versus transurethral resection of the prostate for the large prostate: a prospective nonrandomized bicenter trial with 2-year follow-up. J Endourol. 2008;22:347–54.

Chapter 10
Surgical Treatment: Robotic Simple Prostatectomy

Paulo Afonso de Carvalho and Rafael Ferreira Coelho

10.1 Introduction

Benign prostatic hyperplasia (BPH) is the most common cause of lower urinary tract symptoms (LUTS) and bladder outlet obstruction (BOO) in men. The global incidence and prevalence of this pathology has increased in the past two decades. In the United States, at least 6.5 million men suffer from BPH and it has been estimated that about 1.1 billion men will be affected by 2018 around the world [1–4].

Despite recent advances in the endourological management of BPH, the treatment of LUTS caused by large prostatic adenoma (>100 g) remains a challenge. Currently, open simple prostatectomy (OSP) remains the standard treatment in this particular situation [5–6], providing not only long-term improvement of LUTS, urinary flow, quality of life (QOL), International Prostate Symptom Score (IPSS), but also decreasing post-void residual (PVR) bladder volumes and offering lower reoperation rates when compared with endoscopic treatments. Surgical techniques commonly used are the Freyer [7] (transvesical approach) or Millin procedures [8] (transcapsular approach), both with acceptable results. However, OSP has also been associated with high rates of urosepsis, reoperation, perioperative transfusion and prolonged length of hospital stay [9–11].

In 2002, Mariano et al. [12] described the laparoscopic simple prostatectomy (LSP) technique, combining the benefits of OSP with the potential advantages of a minimally invasive approach, such as decreased blood loss, shorter hospital stay, reduced postoperative pain and a shorter recovery time.

Years later in 2008, Sotelo et al. [13] published the first series of robotic-assisted simple prostatectomy (RASP), describing seven patients undergoing suprapubic transperitoneal transvesical approach with reasonable outcomes. Although attractive, the RASP was classified as an experimental procedure in 2010 by the American Urological Association (AUA) [5], considering that there were insufficient data on which to base treatment recommendations [5, 14].

P.A. de Carvalho (✉) • R.F. Coelho
University of São Paulo School of Medicine, São Paulo, Brazil
e-mail: drpacarvalho@gmail.com; coelhouro@yahoo.com.br

© Springer International Publishing AG 2018
V. Kasivisvanathan, B. Challacombe (eds.), *The Big Prostate*,
https://doi.org/10.1007/978-3-319-64704-3_10

Since then, additional series of RASP have been described in the literature and the procedure is being more commonly performed in men suffering from significant LUTS associated with large prostates.

10.2 Objective

This chapter aims to describe robotic-assisted simple prostatectomy, the perioperative outcomes and its role in the treatment of BPH.

10.3 Indications

The current indications of RASP are similar to traditional indications of open simple prostatectomy [15]:

- Large prostate (over 100 g);
- Acute urinary retention;
- Bladder outlet obstruction refractory to medical therapy;
- Bladder outlet obstruction with diverticulum;
- Recurrent hematuria due to BPH;
- Upper tract changes secondary to BOO;
- Bladder calculi.

10.4 Surgical Technique

The use of robotic technology for prostate surgery is well established in radical prostatectomy. It offers the additional advantages of magnified binocular three-dimensional visualization, motion scaling with tremor filtration, improved surgical ergonomics and miniature wristed articulating instruments with seven degrees of freedom. Those benefits can be also extrapolated to RASP.

Below we describe the main steps of transperitoneal RASP; tips and tricks based on our personal experience are highlighted.

10.5 Patient Position and Port Placement

After induction of general anesthesia, the patient is placed in lithotomy position at a steep Trendelenburg angle with padding of pressure points, identical to a RARP procedure. We use a bean bag for adequate patient positioning and fixation to the surgical table (Fig. 10.1).

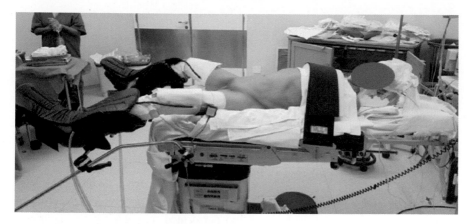

Fig. 10.1 Patient position on the table

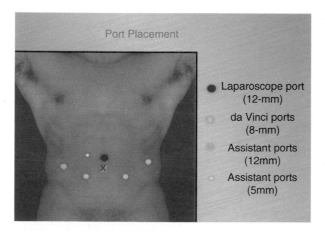

Fig. 10.2 Port placement for RASP procedure

A 18 Fr Foley catheter is inserted into the bladder and 6 ports are placed across the lower abdomen: typically a camera port just above the umbilical scar, three 8-mm arm ports, a 12-mm assistant port in the right flank and a 5 mm for the suction in the right upper quadrant (Fig. 10.2).

10.6   Dissection of the Retzius Space and Apical Dissection

The anterior peritoneum is incised; the dissection progress laterally to the level of the vas deferens bilaterally. After this, the fat over the prostate and prostate-vesical junction is dissected to expose the bladder neck. The endopelvic fascia is then opened immediately lateral to the reflection of the puboprostatic ligaments bilaterally. The Dorsal Venous Complex (DVC) is ligated using a 12-in monofilament polyglytone suture on a CT-1 needle [15, 16]. These last two steps are not essential and the surgery may be performed safely without them [17]. However, in our personal experience DVC ligation appears to decrease bleeding during the anterior dissection of the adenoma without compromising functional outcomes.

10.7   Prostate Adenoma Access

The prostate adenoma may be accessed in different ways. We prefer to perform a 1–2.5 cm transverse incision in the anterior vesicoprostatic junction [17, 18], similar to the anterior bladder neck dissection performed in a RARP; this approach allows easy identification of the plane between the adenoma and the surgical capsule of the prostate without injuring the urethral sphincter and the neurovascular bundle (Fig. 10.3). Another approach is the transvesical technique which can be performed through a proximal horizontal cystostomy [13, 18]. A vertical cystostomy at the dome of the bladder [19] or a midline incision across the prostatic capsule and bladder neck can also be performed [12]. In all the described situations, a good exposure of the adenoma is obtained and there is no evidence that one technique is superior to the other. The decision on what approach to use is mainly based on the surgeon's personal experience (Fig. 10.4).

10.8   Dissection of Prostate Adenoma

We usually perform a horizontal incision at the level of the anterior bladder neck. The plane between the adenoma and the prostatic capsule is then identified and incised over the posterior bladder neck; the adenoma is dissected using a

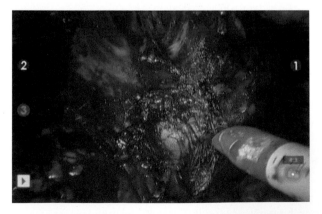

Fig. 10.3 Transverse incision in the anterior vesicoprostatic junction, with easy identification of the adenoma

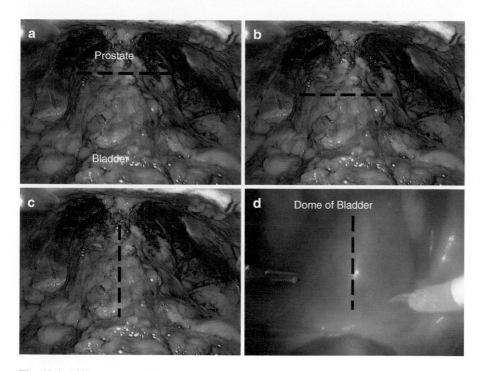

Fig. 10.4 Different approaches to access the prostate adenoma: (**a**) transcapsular, (**b**) horizontal cystostomy, (**c**) midline incision across the prostatic capsule and bladder neck and (**d**) vertical cystostomy at the dome of the bladder (transperitoneal view)

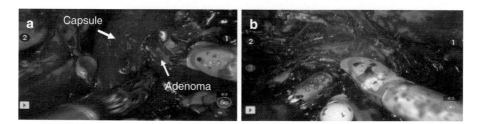

Fig. 10.5 Prostatic adenoma being dissected laterally (**a**) and anteriorly (**b**)

combination of cautery and blunt dissection. This dissection should start posteriorly, preventing blood spillage from the anterior dissection into the posterior plane. The adenoma is then mobilized from the capsule anteriorly and laterally (Fig. 10.5). A 0-Vicryl stay suture can be used for counter traction of the prostate adenoma during the dissection. Finally, the prostatic urethra is carefully transected, avoiding injury to the urinary sphincter, and the adenoma finally is removed (Fig. 10.6). Two 2-0 monocryl sutures are placed at 5 and 7 o'clock positions in the vesicoprostatic junction for additional hemostasis. Hemostasis is revised and bleeding vessels are cauterized or ligated with absorbable sutures.

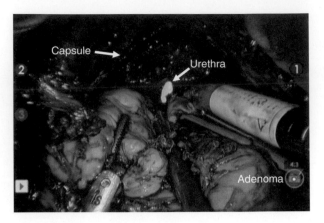

Fig. 10.6 Prostate adenoma being removed after section of the prostatic urethra

10.9 Reconstruction: Advancement of the Bladder Neck Mucosa/Vesico-urethral Anastomosis

In the classical "trigonization" technique the mucosa of the posterior bladder neck is then advanced to the distal urethral mucosa using two figure-of eight 2-0 Vicryl sutures or using a continuous 3-0 monocryl suture [20]. The idea is to reapproximate the mucosa in order to reconstruct the anatomy of the prostatic fossa and promote hemostasis. We have recently described a modified reconstruction technique [16] which includes three surgical steps: plication of the posterior prostatic capsule, modified van Velthoven continuous vesico-urethral anastomosis and suture of the anterior prostatic capsule to the anterior bladder wall. In this approach, after the resection of the adenoma, the posterior capsule is plicated using two 12.5 cm 3-0 monocryl sutures (on RB 1 needles) tied together. The proximal edge of the capsule is approximated to the distal capsule using one arm of the continuous suture. The posterior bladder neck is then sutured to the posterior urethra using the other arm of the suture. A continuous modified van Velthoven vesico-urethral anastomosis is then performed. Two 20-cm 3-0 monocryl sutures of different colours (on RB 1 needles) are tied together with ten knots to provide a bolster for the anastomosis. The posterior part of the vesico-urethral anastomosis is performed with one arm of the suture, in a clockwise direction, from the 5 to 9 o'clock positions. This step is followed by completion of the anterior anastomosis with the second arm of the suture, in counterclockwise fashion (Fig. 10.7). This modified technique of RASP has potential advantages in our experience: reduced blood loss, lower blood transfusion rates, shorter length of hospital stay and no need for postoperative continuous bladder irrigation.

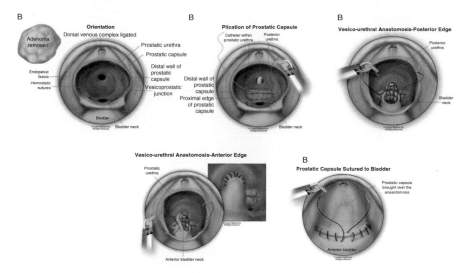

Fig. 10.7 Modified technique of a vesico-urethral anastomosis for RASP procedure

10.10   Closure

A 18F two-way Foley catheter is placed into the bladder and the balloon is inflated with 20 cc of water. Alternatively, a 3 way Foley catheter can be used and the balloon can be insufflated in the prostatic fossa in order to further promote hemostasis; however, with our technique the prostatic fossa is totally plicated and reconstructed precluding the need of this maneuver and the use of three way catheters. A Jackson-Pratt drain is placed into the rectovesical pouch. The midline camera port incision is extended and the specimen (Fig. 10.8) is extracted using an endobag. The aponeurosis is closed using a 0-Vicryl suture, and the skin is closed using a 4-0 Monocryl subcuticular suture. We do not use routinely continuous bladder irrigation as the prostatic fossa is "bypassed" by the anastomosis and the patients do not usually present any grade of hematuria in the early postoperative period.

10.11   RASP Outcomes

10.11.1   Perioperative Outcomes

Consistent data comparing outcomes between RASP, LSP and OSP for the treatment of large prostatic adenoma (>100 g) are limited. There are no randomized clinical trial (level 1 evidence). Comparisons of RASP with Holmium Laser

Fig. 10.8 Prostate
adenoma weighing more
than 100g

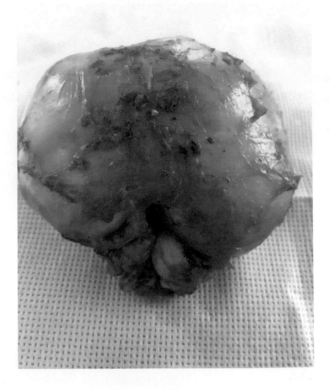

Enucleation of the Prostate (HoLEP) or other endoscopic procedures are also lacking. The main evidence comes from two meta-analyses and multiple small case-series. Below we present data from these analyses in terms of operative time, estimated blood loss and transfusion, length of hospital stay, complications, functional outcomes, duration of catheterization and cost comparison.

10.11.2 Operative Time

In a meta-analysis [21] comparing minimally invasive simple prostatectomy (MISP) with OSP, from 27 observational studies published between 2004 and 2014, including 119 RASP cases, the mean operative time was 141 min, about 40 min longer than OSP. This was probably a consequence of different learning curves between both methods [22], as well as potential bias of including the LSP cases. In the largest exclusive RASP series to date, Pokorny [23] obtained a shorter operative time of 97 min (comparable to OSP) with a median preoperative prostate volume of 129 mL (104–180). In our initial series the mean operative time was 90 ± 17.6 min

(75-120 min) with a median preoperative prostate volume of 157 mL (90–300) [16], reaffirming the importance of being familiar with the robotic technique.

10.12 Estimated Blood Loss and Transfusion

Although OSP is a generally safe procedure, it is often associated with relatively high rates of perioperative transfusion. Early RASP case series also reported high estimated blood loss (EBL), with a mean of 558 mL (150–1125 mL) in one of the early publications [24]. However, results have improved over time and RASP case series after 2008 report a mean operative blood loss of 183 mL and low transfusion rates ranging from 0 to 5% [25]; these transfusion rates are significantly lower than the 17% transfusion rates observed in OSP cases from the recent US Nationwide Inpatient Sample (NIS) [26]. This same study, using an adjusted transfusion prevalence, revealed a 50% lower transfusion rate for MISP but this difference did not quite reach statistical significance (odds ratio 0.47; 95% CI, 0.18–1.26). In another recent meta-analysis, Banapour et al. [18], reporting 109 RASP cases from eight non-comparative case series, showed a mean operative blood loss of 197 mL with a transfusion rate of 0%, adding further supportive data that RASP is associated with less blood loss and perioperative transfusion when compared to OSP.

In our series [16], the modified vesico-urethral anastomosis technique in RASP assures low EBL and low transfusion rates, with the mean EBL of 208 ± 66 (100–300) mL with a transfusion rate of 0%, in a reproducible and safe method.

Although RCTs are lacking at this time, data suggests that robotic assisted surgery leads to less bleeding and less perioperative transfusion rates.

10.13 Length of Hospital of Stay

In the NIS series, studying 6027 OSP cases and 182 MISP cases, the median stay for MISP was 2 days shorter than for OSP (2 vs. 4 days). However, this was not statistically significant (p = 0.19) probably because the analysis was underpowered [26]. In consistent RASP series, Pokorny [23] and Autorino [27] respectively showed a median length of stay of 4 days (3–5 days) and 2 days (1–4 days). In a meta-analysis [21], evaluating some case series, the length of hospital stay was significantly shorter in MISP group with 1.6 days, (95% CI: 0.2–2.9, p = 0.02) compared with OSP group with 7.6 days.

As described above, our technique can reduce the length of hospital stay by eliminating the need for postoperative bladder irrigation, with a median stay of 1 day, we have demonstrated that shorter hospital stay is possible with RASP [16].

10.13.1 Complications

Due to the variability in the methods of reporting and classifying complications, the comparison of complication rates between different series and techniques is a difficult [25], since not all papers comply with all the Martin criteria [28] for the description of postoperative complications.

In the systematic review about the issue, Lucca [21] summarizes the current data on perioperative complications (n = 114). Overall, there were no significant differences between OSP and MISP groups (OR 0.64, 95% CI 0.4–1.03, p = 0.066), as well as for each individual complication: blood transfusion (OR 0.54, 95% CI: 0.13–2.10, p = 0.386), urinary retention (OR 0.93, 95% CI: 0.39–2.15, p = 0.867), urinary tract infection (OR 0.61, 95% CI: 0.07–5.66, p = 0.066) and Re-operation (OR 1.82, 95% CI: 0.48–6.20, p = 0.382); note that this analysis is not exclusively with RASP cases as it includes also LSP.

Autorino et al. [27], evaluating 1330 MISP cases, report a low postoperative complication rate and that most of the complications in 90 days were low grade Clavien 1–2 (8.8%), which translates into minimal clinical impact on the regular postoperative course. This data supports lower complication rates than those typically seen with OSP.

In unpublished data [33], comparing HoLEP (45 cases) versus RASP (81 cases) similar complication rates with no Clavien >3 grade were found in both groups (p = 0.7).

Overall, there is a need for prospective well-designed studies to adequately assess for true differences in complication rates between different modalities.

10.14 Duration of Catheterization

Some evidence indicates that there is no difference in catheterization time between RASP and OSP [13, 16, 17, 18, 19, 23, 24]. On the other hand, a meta-analysis comparing MISP and OSP noted decreased catheter duration for MISP (weighted mean difference −1.3 days, 95% CI: 2.5 to −0.06, p = 0.04) [21]; however, the criteria for removing the catheter were not clearly stated and most likely not uniform across the different series and surgical approaches.

When RASP is compared with HoLEP the catheterization time was shorter for HoLEP group (2 vs. 4 days; p = 0.0001), however, the two groups were not statistically similar to each other [33].

In our experience, the modified technique of robotic–assisted simple prostatectomy allows a safe withdrawal of catheter at an average of 4.8 days. A cystogram is performed in all patients on postoperative day 4–6. Up to 200 mL contrast medium is instilled into the bladder under gravity. In the early publication of our modified technique, no leakage was observed [16].

To the date no substantial difference between catheter durations has been demonstrated in published RASP and OSP studies [25].

10.15   Functional Outcomes

Perioperative and short-term functional data seem similar in RASP and OSP. A retrospective study presented data about 67 RASP cases and demonstrated improvement in functional outcomes ($p < 0.001$) at a follow-up of 6 months [2–12], with a postoperative Qmax of 23 mL/s [16–35], IPSS of 3 points (0–8) and post-void residual volume of 0 mL (0–36) [23]. A meta-analysis [21] comparing MISP (including RASP cases) with OSP reported an average aggregate improvement in the maximum urinary flow rate (Qmax) of 14.3 mL/s and IPSS improvement of 17.2 points for MISP (n = 163 patients), similar to data obtained by OSP (n = 252), but the small study size, publications bias and short follow-up are limitations.

Assessing RASP versus HoLEP, both groups showed respectively an improvement of maximum flow rate (+15 vs. +11 mL/s, p = 0.7), a reduction of post-void residual (73 vs. 100 mL, p = 0.4) and improvement in IPSS (−20 vs. −18, p = 0.8) with median follow-up of 12 months in the RASP group and 5 months in the HoLEP group [33].

Using a modified technique of robotic simple prostatectomy, we obtained a significant improvement from baseline in IPSS (average preoperative vs. postoperative, 19.8 ± 9.6 vs. 5.5 ± 2.5, p = 0.01), a mean maximum urine flow (average preoperative vs. postoperative 7.75 ± 3.3 vs. 19 ± 4.5 mL/s, p = 0.019) at 2 months after RASP and all patients were continent (defined as the use of no pads) at 2 months after RASP [16]. It is important to note that no other available study reported the continence rate in its postoperative period.

Overall, these three approaches showed no differences in perioperative complication rates and consistent improvement in functional outcomes in the short to medium term [18, 26, 33], but long-term results are needed.

10.15.1   Learning Curve

Currently no papers evaluating the RASP learning curve have been published. Existing data tends to be reported by experienced surgeons. RASP using a modified technique of vesico-urethral anastomosis certainly requires a certain mastery of robotic technology, however for those surgeons who are accustomed to performing RARP, this learning is simple and safe. Therefore, we envisage that for surgeons with existing expertise in RARP, few cases in RASP are necessary to achieve reproducible and adequate results.

10.15.2 Cost Comparison

Costs related to minimally invasive technologies, especially robotic technology, remain a highly debated issue [34]. A formal cost analysis is difficult given the fact that hospital costs and reimbursement issues vary significantly between countries and healthcare systems. Certainly the high upfront and maintenance costs of a robot mean that this technology is not easily accessible to many Urological centres. However if the robot is already in place for other types of surgery then the relative costs are much reduced.

Matei [35] reported a cost of €3840 per RASP versus more than €5000 for OSP with the higher costs of OSP being due to higher hospitalization costs. They also showed that cost of bipolar transurethral resection of the prostate in the very large prostate was similar to that of RASP. TURP in the very large prostate may of course require more than one procedure and inpatient stay which may explain these findings. However, Sutherland [17] reported that the cost of RASP was higher than OSP, adding an average of $2797 to the operating charges. In this context future research should adjust the time-horizon for cost-effectiveness analyses to account for costs associated with complications, transfusion rates and hospital length of stay. Certainly the arrival of cheaper robotic systems is eagerly anticipated and may tip the cost-effectiveness ratio in favour of RASP for the very large prostate.

10.15.3 Conclusions

RASP appears to be an effective and safe treatment option for men with symptomatic BPH and large prostates (>100 g). Although prospective randomized trials comparing RASP to other treatment modalities are lacking, existing comparative series would suggest that improvements in Qmax and IPSS are similar to those of OSP. RASP may also offer lower rates of perioperative transfusion and shorter hospital admissions than OSP. Certainly, in institutions with access to the robot and where appropriate expertise in robotic pelvic surgery is available, RASP should be considered as an important treatment option for the symptomatic large prostate.

References

1. Wei JT, Calhoun E, Jacobsen SJ. Urologic diseases in America project: benign prostatic hyperplasia. J Urol. 2008;179:S75–80.
2. Irwin DE, Kopp ZS, Agatep B, Milsom I, Abrams P. Worldwide prevalence estimates of lower urinary tract symptoms, overactive bladder, urinary incontinence and bladder outlet obstruction. BJU Int. 2011;108:1132–8.

3. Kupelian V, Fitzgerald MP, Kaplan SA, Norgaard JP, Chiu GR, Rosen RC. Association of nocturia and mortality: results from the Third National Health and Nutrition Examination Survey.
J Urol. 2011;185:571–7.
4. Groves HK, Chang D, Palazzi K, Cohen S, Parsons JK. The incidence of acute urinary retention secondary to BPH is increasing among California men. Prostate Cancer Prostatic Dis.
2013;16:260–5.
5. McVary KT, Roehrborn CG, Avins AL, Barry MJ, Bruskewitz RC, Donnell RF, et al. Update
on AUA guideline on the management of the benign prostatic hyperplasia. J Urol.
2011;185:1793–803.
6. Oelke M, Bachmann A, Descazeaud A, Emberton M, Gravas S, Michel MC, et al. EAU guidelines on treatment and follow-up of the non-neurogenic male lower urinary tract symptoms including benign prostatic obstruction. Eur Urol. 2013;63:118–40.
7. Freyer PJ. One thousand cases of total enucleation of the prostate for radical cure of enlargement of that organ. Br Med J. 1912;2:868–70.
8. Millin R. Retropubic prostatectomy: new extravesical technique: report on 20 cases. Lancet.
1945;2:693–6.
9. Serretta V, Morgia G, Fondacaro L, Curto G, Lo Bianco A, Pirritano D, et al. Open prostatectomy for benign prostatic enlargement in Southern Europe in the late 1900s: a contemporary series of the 1800 interventions. Urology. 2002;60(4):623–7.
10. Gratzke C, Schlenker B, Seitz M, Karl A, Hermanek P, Lack N, et al. Complications and early
postoperative outcome after open prostatectomy in patients with benign prostatic enlargement:
results of a prospective multicenter study. J Urol. 2007;177(4):1419–22.
11. Suer E, Gokce I, Yaman O, Anafarta K, Göğüş O. Open prostatectomy is still a valid option for
the large prostates: a high-volume, single-center experience. Urology. 2008;72(1):90–4.
12. Mariano MB, Graziottin TM, Tefilli MV. Laparoscopic prostatectomy with vascular control for
benign prostatic hyperplasia. J Urol. 2002;167:2528–9.
13. Sotelo R, Clavijo R, Carmona O, Garcia A, Banda E, Miranda M, et al. Robotic simple prostatectomy. J Urol. 2008;179:513–5.
14. Parsons JK, Patel ND. Robotic-assisted simple prostatectomy: Is there evidence to go beyond
the experimental stage? Curr Urol Rep. 2014;15:443–7.
15. Patel MN, Hemal AK. Robot-assisted laparoscopic simple anatomic prostatectomy. Urol Clin
North Am. 2014;41(4):485–92.
16. Coelho RF, Chauhan S, Sivaraman A, Palmer KJ, Orvieto MA, Rocco B, et al. Modified technique of robotic-assisted simple prostatectomy: advantages of a vesico-urethral anastomosis. BJUI. 2011;109:426–33.
17. Sutherland DE, Perez DS, Weeks DC. Robot-assisted simple prostatectomy for severe benign
prostatic hyperplasia. J Endourol. 2011;25:641–4.
18. Banapour P, Patel N, Kane CJ, Cohen SA, Parsons JK. Robotic-assisted simple prostatectomy:
a systematic review and report of a single institution case series. Prostate Cancer Prostatic
Dis. 2014;17:1–5.
19. Leslie S, Abreu AL, Chopra S, Ramos P, Park D, Berger AK, et al. Transvesical robotic simple
prostatectomy: initial clinical experience. Eur Urol. 2014;66(2):321–9.
20. Dubey D, Hemal AK. Robotic-assisted simple prostatectomy with complete urethrovesical
reconstruction. Indian J Urol. 2012;28(2):231–2.
21. Lucca IH, Shariat S, Hofbauer S, Klatte T. Outcomes of minimally invasive simple prostatectomy for benign prostatic hyperplasia: a systematic review and meta-analysis. World J Urol.
2015;33:563–70.
22. Abboudi H, Khan MS, Guru KA, Froghi S, de Win G, Van Poppel H et al. Learning curves for
urological procedures: a systematic review. BJU Int 2013;114(4):617–29.
23. Pokorny M, Novara G, Geurts N, Dovey Z, Groote R, Ploumidis A, et al. Robot-assisted simple
prostatectomy for treatment of lower urinary tract symptoms secondary to benign prostatic enlargement: surgical technique and outcomes in a high-volume robotic centre. Eur
Urol. 2015;68:451–7.

24. Yuh B, Laungani R, Perlmutter A, Eun D, Peabody JO, Mohler JL, et al. Robot-assisted Millin's retropubic prostatectomy: case series. Can J Urol. 2008;15:4101–5.
25. Holden M, Parsons JK. Robotic-assisted simple prostatectomy: an overview. Urol Clin North Am. 2016;43(3):385–91.
26. Parsons JK, Rangarajan S, Palazzi K, Chang D. A national, comparative analysis of perioperative outcomes of open and minimally invasive simple prostatectomy. J Endourol. 2015;29:919–24.
27. Autorino R, Zargar H, Mariano MB, Sanchez-Salas R, Sotelo R, Chlosta PL, et al. Perioperative outcomes of robotic and laparoscopic simple prostatectomy: a European-American Multi-institucional analysis. Eur Urol. 2015;68:86–94.
28. Martin RC 2nd, Brennan MF, Jaques DP. Quality of complication reporting in the surgical literature. Ann Surg. 2002;235:803–13.
29. Porpiglia F, Terrone C, Renard J, Grande S, Musso F, Cossu M, et al. Transcapsular adenomectomy (Millin): a comparative study, extraperitoneal laparoscopy versus open surgery. Eur Urol. 2006;49(1):120–6.
30. McCullough TC, Heldwein FL, Soon SJ, Galiano M, Barret E, Cathelineau X, et al. Laparoscopic versus open simple prostatectomy: an evaluation of morbidity. J Endourol. 2009;23(1):129–33.
31. Baumert H, Ballaro A, Dugardin F, Kaisary AV. Laparoscopic versus open simple prostatectomy: a comparative study. J Urol. 2006;175(5):1691–4.
32. Garcia-Segui A, Gascón-Mir M. Comparative study between laparoscopic extraperitoneal and open adenomectomy. Actas Urol Esp. 2012;36(2):110–6.
33. Umari P, Fossati N, Gandaglia G, Pokorny M, Groot RD, Geurts N, et al. Robotic Assisted Simple Prostatectomy (RASP) versus Holmium Laser Enucleation of the Prostate (HoLEP) for lower urinary tract symptoms in patients with large prostate (>100mL): a comparative analysis from a high-volume center. J Urol 2016;197(4):1108–14.
34. Ahmed K, Ibrahim A, Wang TT, Khan N, Challacombe B, Khan MS, et al. Assessing the cost effectiveness of robotics in urological surgery—a systematic review. BJU Int. 2012;110:1544–56.
35. Matei DV, Brascia A, Mazzoleni F, Spinelli M, Musi G, Melegari S, et al. Robotic-assisted simple prostatectomy (RASP): does it make sense? BJU Int. 2012;110:E972–9.

Chapter 11
Open Simple Prostatectomy

Manmeet Saluja, Jonathan Masters, and Simon Van Rij

11.1 Introduction

A book on the management of the large prostate would not be complete without a chapter on the operation that started it all; the open simple prostatectomy. Some may say that this is a procedure destined for the history books, yet still today it is commonly performed in many countries around the world.

First popularised by Freyer over 100 years ago, this operation developed into the gold standard for the surgical treatment of men with symptomatic Benign Prostatic Hyperplasia (BPH) [1]. Two key approaches have been described for this procedure: the transvesical (Freyer's) approach or the retropubic (Millin's) [2] approach. Each technique has both advantages and disadvantages which will be discussed in detail. Open Prostatectomy remains a recommended surgical technique for men with large prostates requiring surgery in all the major urological guidelines [3]. It is often used as the benchmark to compare any new technique for surgical outcomes. Therefore, surgeons dealing with BPH still need to be aware of the technique and when it may be required.

There is marked variation worldwide in the percentage of BPH surgery still undertaken via the open technique. In a recent survey [4], 78% of Urologists were still performing Open Prostatectomy in their practice. This was independent of surgeon age and year of residency completion. However, open prostatectomy accounted for only 0.1% of all BPH surgery in USA [5] with a notable decreasing trend over the last 10 years [6] (see Fig. 11.1). This is likely due to the diffusion of endoscopic techniques; particularly those involving enucleation principles. In Europe, the prevalence of open prostatectomy as surgical treatment for BPH is as high as 14% in France, 32% in Italy and 40% in Israel [7]. Rates of 15–40% [8] have been reported from the developing countries; however this may an underestimate due to less published research from the developing world.

This chapter will present the place of open prostatectomy in the modern day urology practice.

M. Saluja (✉) • J. Masters • S. Van Rij
Auckland Hospital, Auckland, New Zealand
e-mail: manmeet.saluja@gmail.com; mjgmasters@gmail.com; simonvanrij@gmail.com

© Springer International Publishing AG 2018
V. Kasivisvanathan, B. Challacombe (eds.), *The Big Prostate*,
https://doi.org/10.1007/978-3-319-64704-3_11

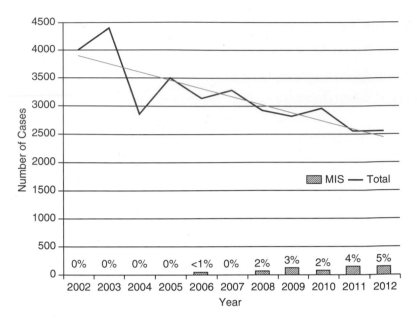

Fig. 11.1 Trend of simple prostatectomies between 2002 and 2012 in USA—open and minimally invasive (MIS) (Pariser et al. 2015) [6]

11.2 Indications

Open simple prostatectomy has been typically described for benign prostatic hyperplasia measuring greater than 80–100 g^{gm}. Other indications include patients with large bladder calculi or symptomatic bladder diverticulae, which could be removed at the same time as the enucleation. Some patients may not be a candidate for endoscopic surgery (for example: if they are at high risk of recurrent urethral strictures or their large prostate or body size prohibits the entry of the scope into the bladder). Similarly, patients who are unable to be placed in a dorsal lithotomy position may benefit from an open approach [12]. Contraindications include patients with known prostate cancer, presence of a small gland and previous pelvic surgery or radiation.

11.3 Pre-op Evaluation

Patients need a comprehensive history and examination with assessment of their PSA and renal function. TRUS or MRI can be used to establish prostate size [33]. If the patient has recurrent UTI, haematuria or deranged renal function, the upper tracts need to be evaluated with either a CT or Ultrasound.

11.4   Operative Techniques

The retropubic approach offers direct visualization of the prostate with minimal trauma to the bladder [2]. However, it may make excision of a diverticulum, removal of calculi or excision of large median lobes difficult. In contrast, the suprapubic approach may compromise hemostasis as direct visualization of the prostatic fossa is reduced. Perineal prostatectomy is rarely used and lacks robust data but may be useful in morbidly obese patients [21].

11.5   Retropubic Prostatectomy

Under a general or a spinal anesthetic, patients are positioned supine in a modern Trendelenburg position with ASIS positioned over the kidney rest. A large urethral catheter is placed and the balloon is inflated with 30 mL. Either a low midline or a Pfannsteil incision is performed and dissection is performed to enter the space of Retzius. A Bookwalter® retractor with a middle blade is used. The pre-prostatic fat is swept away in an up and down direction [22] and the superficial branch of DVC diathermied.

Pre-emptive hemostasis is a key aspect of the operation and has been described in many different methods. One measure is to control the DVC after incising the endopelvic fascia in a similar way to a radical prostatectomy [12].

Another approach is to initially place a suture as far laterally on each side of the prostate (Fig. 11.2). Transverse tramline sutures with a 5 mm gap between are then applied on each side of the incision line on the prostate (Fig. 11.2). Each stitch interlocks with the neighbouring suture and the row of sutures finish at the previously placed lateral sutures. These sutures reduce bleeding as they control the capsular veins and stop the capsule from tearing during enucleation. A transverse

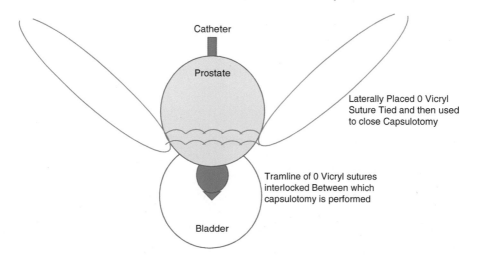

Fig. 11.2 Technique of tramline sutures to achieve hemostasis during retropubic prostatectomy

incision is then performed between the tramline sutures (1 cm caudal to the bladder neck) to the lateral limits of capsular incision.

The prostate adenoma is then enucleated. The plane between the adenoma and the prostatic capsule is opened up by spreading scissors underneath the capsule. A finger is then swept side to side and posteriorly. Scissors are used to incise the anterior commissure from bladder neck to the apex [12]. Any adhesions between the adenoma and the capsule are then dissected sharply. A pinch action is used to remove the adenoma off the urethral mucosa and the bladder neck trigonalised. The median lobe is teased out and any bladder stones can be removed at this point with finger or sponge holder (Fig. 11.3).

Once complete enucelation is performed, the lateral sutures are used to close the incision. If ongoing bleeding, sutures can be placed at the bladder neck at the 5 and 7 o'clock position [12] ensuring to avoid the ureteric orifi bilaterally. The indwelling urethral catheter is then place on irrigation as soon as the capsule closed. A retropubic drain is inserted and placed on low suction (Fig. 11.4).

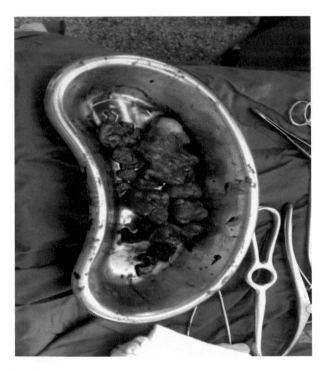

Fig. 11.3 Enucleated prostate specimen

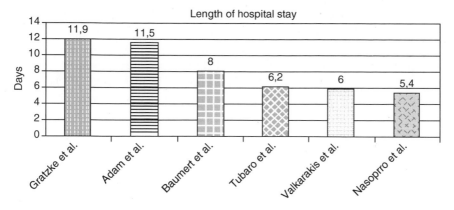

Fig. 11.4 Length of hospital stay (Modified from Gratzke et al. 2007) [29]

11.6   Suprapubic Prostatectomy

A urethral catheter is placed and the bladder filled with 300 mL normal saline. Once exposure is gained into the retropubic space, a transverse cystotomy is performed between two stay sutures. Bilateral ureteric orifi are identified. Any calculi are removed at this stage. Retractors are placed and a malleable blade is used to retract the bladder superiorly and expose the trigone.

Preventive hemostatic measures include controlling the DVC or temporary hypogastric artery ligation [23]. A circular incision is performed through the bladder mucosa around the prostate avoiding the trigone. A finger is inserted into the prostatic fossa cracking the anterior commissure. The plane between the prostatic adenoma and pseudo-capsule is then developed circumferentially. A pinch action is used at the apex to avoid excess traction so as not to avulse the urethra and injure the sphincter. Any adhesions can be cut or diathermied, however if there is unusual adherence then cancer should be suspected [24].

Hemostasis is achieved by placing a gauze pack into the prostatic fossa. Figure of eight sutures are placed at the 5 and 7 o'clock position at the bladder neck. Prostatic fossa bleeders can be over sewed specifically if needed. For ongoing bleeding, Malament [25] has described placing a 1-0 nylon purse string suture around the vesical neck and bring it out through the abdominal skin and tying it down firmly. These sutures can be cut day 2–3 post operatively. O'Connor [26] has described attaining hemostasis by creating capsular tamponade by the use of capsular plication on each side of the fossa. Other methods include placing oxidized cellulose (Surgicel©) in the fossa [27]˙ An IDC is inserted and irrigation initiated once the bladder mucosa is sutured. A suprapubic catheter may also be inserted but is usually not necessary. The second layer of bladder closure is then performed. Hematuria can usually be managed by temporary catheter traction.

11.7   Post-operative Management

Continuous bladder irrigation is titrated post-operatively. If the catheter is placed on traction, this needs to be released within 12 h [24]. Patient is ambulated, analgesia given and thrombo-prophylaxis addressed cautiously. Drain is removed when drainage amount reduces and the catheter can be removed on day 3–5 with or without a cystogram prior.

11.8   Outcomes and Complications

Current evidence regarding outcomes from Open Prostatectomy mainly stems from historical data or from trials where Open Prostatectomy was used as the control arm for the evaluation of newer techniques. Repeatedly, it has been proven to provide a maximal and sustainable benefit to patient's symptoms. Mean flow rates are increased by up to 20 mL/s and mean IPPS scores decreased by up to 19 points [38] (Table 11.1). Furthermore, most studies fail to report the rates of freedom from

Table 11.1 Outcomes of open prostatectomy

	Suer et al. (2008)	Gratzke et al. (2007)	Tubaro et al. (2001)	Carneiro et al. (2016)	Varkarakis et al. (2004)	Naspro et al. (2006)[b]
Mean weight (g)	88.7	84.8	63	Not recorded	Not recorded	87.90
Operative time (min)	Not recorded	81	62.5	126	Not recorded	58.31
Flow rate increase (mL/s)	14.4	12.4	19.8	15.4	16.2	11.79
Decrease in PVR (mL)	88	128	124	Not recorded	104.1	Not recorded
Decrease in IPSS	11.1	Not recorded	18.5	19.52	23.3	9.4
Hospital Stay	6.74	11.9	6.2	4.6	6	5.4
UTI %	Not recorded	5.1	12.5	7	2.6	Not recorded
Blood Transfusion %	12.7	7.5	0	3.9	6.8	17.9
Incontinence %	0.7	Not recorded	Not recorded	4[a]	0	11
Mortality %	0.003	0.2	0	0	0	Not recorded
Surgical revision %	4.8	3.7	6.25	7	3.9	5.7

[a]Early UTI
[b]24 month follow-up

catheterization for those men who were catheter dependent prior to surgery [8]. Anecdotally within our own institution, men with extremely large prostates who are catheter dependent are often the strongest indicator for open surgery due to the high success rate of ending up without a long term catheter.

Open prostatectomy has been classically associated with a transfusion rate of 3–10% [8, 28] (Table 11.1). However with improved surgical technique and better postoperative management, these rates are improved nowadays [29]. Post-operative UTI has been reported in 3–17% of cases [29] and wound infection in 2–4% [30]. Reported rates of early and late urinary incontinence were 3.7% and 1.2%, respectively [31]. In the longer term, patients may experience erectile dysfunction in 3–5% of cases and nearly all have retrograde ejaculation. Bladder neck contracture can present in 2–5% of cases [28, 32]. Ostetitis pubis is rare but usually presents 4–6 weeks post operatively with pubic pain and low-grade fever and usually improves with anti-inflammatory drugs. These low rates of complication are very comparable to other surgical techniques.

11.9 Open Prostatectomy Compared to Other Techniques

There are numerous modern trials comparing different surgical techniques with Open Prostatectomy. Referenced in this section are the important trials along with pertinent outcomes when compared to open prostatectomy.

11.9.1 vs. Monopolar TURP

Compared to TURP, open prostatectomy offers a lower re-treatment rate (1.8–4.5% vs. 12–15% respectively) [9–12], larger volume of prostate removal and avoids the risk of TURP syndrome in large glands. However there is increased length of stay, postoperative pain and increased risk of hemorrhage with open surgery [8, 11].

11.9.2 vs. Bipolar TURP

Multiple prospective RCT's have shown Bipolar TURP with Normal Saline irrigation has advantage over monopolar TURP's as it reduces bleeding and risk of TURP syndrome [38]. However, there are limited head to head trials comparing it to open prostatectomy for large glands. One randomized trial reported Bipolar TURP to have similar functional surgical outcomes and improvement in flow rates and PVR's [36]. However bleeding, lengths of stay and retreatment rates were better in the Bipolar group [39].

11.9.3   vs. Bipolar Electrosurgical Enucleation

A metanalysis of 4 RCT's comparing Bipolar enucleation to Open Prostatectomy was recently performed [35]. Bipolar enucleation offers a reduced haemoglobin decrease (by 1.22 g/dL), shorter catheterisation time (by 3.78 days) and hospital stay (by 4.43 days). Qmax, IPSS, QOL, PVR and IIE-5 scores were similar after at least a year of follow up [19, 20]. Bipolar enucleation yields a smaller measured prostatic resection (by 8gm) but this may be due to effect of vaporisation and is unlikely to be clinically significant [35].

11.9.4   vs. HOLEP

There have been three RCT's published comparing Open Prostatectomy vs. HOLEP [15, 16, 34]. A meta-analysis of these showed HOLEP resulted in less blood loss (by 0.95 g/dL) and a shorter hospital stay (by 5.84 days) but was associated with a longer operative time (by 32 min) [35]. Resection weight, peak flow rates, residual volumes, IPSS scores and overall complication rate were similar between both groups even after five years of follow up [16]. Despite this a prolonged learning curve has limited its uptake around the world [35].

11.9.5   vs. Photoselective Vaporization of the Prostate (PVP)

There is an increasing use of PVP for large size prostate glands; however data comparing with Open Prostatectomy are limited. Non randomised studies suggest the Greenlight PVP may be safe in patients with prostate sizes >80 g and equally efficacious compared to smaller glands [17, 18]. However, one study showed a higher conversion rate to a TURP (8.4%) due to bleeding [37]. Further prospective trials are therefore needed to establish its role in the management of large prostates.

11.9.6   vs. Laparoscopic and Robotic Surgery

Laparoscopic/Robotic surgery can provide better hemostasis, transfusion rates and shorter hospital stay, however is associated with a difficult learning curve, significantly increased cost and longer operative time [13, 14].

11.10   Conclusion

Open prostatectomy still has a relevant role in management of BPH, particularly for very large prostates over 100 g. It is efficacious and has durable outcomes; however its use is limited due to associated morbidity and advent of newer procedures. Newer data is required to reflect the current day outcomes especially from developing countries, where the procedure is still widely used. For selected patients, this procedure may remain the most appropriate choice for many years to come.

References

1. Fitzpatrick JM. Minimally invasive and endoscopic management of benign prostatic hyperplasia. In: Wein AJ, Kavoussi LR, Nocick AC, editors. Campbell–Walsh urology. 9th ed. Philadelphia: Saunders Elsevier; 2007.
2. Millin T. Retropubic prostatectomy; a new extravesical technique; report of 20 cases. Lancet. 1945;2(6380):693–6.
3. Oelke M, et al. EAU guidelines on the treatment and follow-up of non-neurogenic male lower urinary tract symptoms including benign prostatic obstruction. Eur Urol. 2013;64(1):118–40.
4. Lee NG, Xue H, Lerner LB. Trends and attitudes in surgical management of benign prostatic hyperplasia. Can J Urol. 2012;19(2):6170–5.
5. Black L, et al. An examination of treatment patterns and costs of care among patients with benign prostatic hyperplasia. Am J Manag Care. 2006;12(4 Suppl):S99–S110.
6. Pariser JJ, et al. National trends of simple prostatectomy for benign prostatic hyperplasia with an analysis of risk factors for adverse perioperative outcomes. Urology. 2015;86(4):721–5.
7. Semmens JB, et al. Trends in repeat prostatectomy after surgery for benign prostate disease: application of record linkage to healthcare outcomes. BJU Int. 1999;84(9):972–5.
8. Serretta V, et al. Open prostatectomy for benign prostatic enlargement in southern Europe in the late 1990s: a contemporary series of 1800 interventions. Urology. 2002;60(4):623–7.
9. Mebust WK, et al. Transurethral prostatectomy: immediate and postoperative complications. A cooperative study of 13 participating institutions evaluating 3,885 patients. J Urol. 1989;141(2):243–7.
10. Roos NP, et al. Mortality and reoperation after open and transurethral resection of the prostate for benign prostatic hyperplasia. N Engl J Med. 1989;320(17):1120–4.
11. Simforoosh N, et al. Open prostatectomy versus transurethral resection of the prostate, where are we standing in the new era? A randomized controlled trial. Urol J. 2010;7(4):262–9.
12. Han M, Partin AW. Retropubic and suprapubic open prostatectomy. In: Wein AJ, editor. Campbell-Walsh urology. 10th ed. Philadelphia: Elsevier; 2012. p. 2641–67.
13. Matei, D.V., et al. Robot-assisted simple prostatectomy (RASP): does it make sense? BJU Int. 2012;110(11 Pt C):E972-9.
14. Baumert H, et al. Laparoscopic versus open simple prostatectomy: a comparative study. J Urol. 2006;175(5):1691–4.
15. Naspro R, et al. Holmium laser enucleation of the prostate versus open prostatectomy for prostates >70 g: 24-month follow-up. Eur Urol. 2006;50(3):563–8.

16. Kuntz RM, Lehrich K, Ahyai SA. Holmium laser enucleation of the prostate versus open prostatectomy for prostates greater than 100 grams: 5-year follow-up results of a randomised clinical trial. Eur Urol. 2008;53(1):160–6.

17. Woo H, et al. Outcome of Greenlight HPS 120-W laser therapy in specific patient populations: those in retention, on anticoagulants, and with large prostates ($\geq$ 80ml). European Journal Supplements. 2008;7(4):378–83.

18. Rajbabu K, et al. Photoselective vaporization of the prostate with the potassium-titanyl-phosphate laser in men with prostates of >100 mL. BJU Int. 2007;100(3):593–8.

19. Ou R, et al. Transurethral enucleation and resection of the prostate vs transvesical prostatectomy for prostate volumes >80 mL: a prospective randomized study. BJU Int. 2013;112(2):239–45.

20. Li M, et al. Endoscopic enucleation versus open prostatectomy for treating large benign prostatic hyperplasia: a meta-analysis of randomized controlled trials. PLoS One. 2015;10(3):e0121265.

21. Bernie JE, Schmidt JD. Simple perineal prostatectomy: lessons learned from a modern series. J Urol. 2003. 170(1):115–8; discussion 118.

22. Fitzpatrick JM. Millin retropubic prostatectomy. BJU Int. 2008;102(7):906–16.

23. Yu GW, Miller HC., Suprapubic prostatectomy, critical operative maneuvers in urologic surgery. St. Louis: Mosby; 1996. pp. 199–206.

24. Moddler JK, McVary KT. Suprapubic prostatectomy. In: Smith J, Howards S, Preminger G, editors. Hinman's atlas of urologic surgery. 3rd ed. Philadelphia: Elsevier; 2012.

25. Malament M. Maximal Hemostasis in Suprapubic Prostatectomy. Surg Gynecol Obstet. 1965;120:1307–12.

26. O'Connor, VJ. Suprapubic prostatectomy. Urologic surgery. Philadelphia: JB Lippincott; 1983. pp. 853–60.

27. Ellis JW, Wright JL. Complications of simple prostatectomy. 4 ed. Complications of urologic surgery. Philadelphia: Elsevier; 2010. pp. 497–501.

28. Varkarakis I, et al. Long-term results of open transvesical prostatectomy from a contemporary series of patients. Urology. 2004;64(2):306–10.

29. Gratzke C, et al. Complications and early postoperative outcome after open prostatectomy in patients with benign prostatic enlargement: results of a prospective multicenter study. J Urol. 2007;177(4):1419–22.

30. Condie JD Jr, Cutherell L, Mian A. Suprapubic prostatectomy for benign prostatic hyperplasia in rural Asia: 200 consecutive cases. Urology. 1999;54(6):1012–6.

31. Carneiro A, et al. Open suprapubic versus retropubic prostatectomy in the treatment of benign prostatic hyperplasia during resident's learning curve: a randomized controlled trial. Int Braz J Urol. 2016;42(2):284–92.

32. Tubaro A, et al. A prospective study of the safety and efficacy of suprapubic transvesical prostatectomy in patients with benign prostatic hyperplasia. J Urol. 2001;166(1):172–6.

33. Tewari A, et al. Comparison of transrectal ultrasound prostatic volume estimation with magnetic resonance imaging volume estimation and surgical specimen weight in patients with benign prostatic hyperplasia. J Clin Ultrasound. 1996;24(4):169–74.

34. Zhang Y, et al. Transurethral holmium laser enucleation for prostate adenoma greater than 100 g. Zhonghua Nan Ke Xue. 2007;13:1091–3.

35. Li M, et al. Endoscopic enucleation versus open prostatectomy for treating large benign prostatic hyperplasia: a meta-analysis of randomized controlled trials. PLoS One. 2015;10(3):e0121265.

36. Komura K, et al. Incidence of urethral stricture after bipolar transurethral resection of the prostate using TURis: results from a randomised trial. BJU Int. 2015;115(4):644–52.

37. Hueber PA, et al. Photoselective vaporization of the prostate for benign prostatic hyperplasia using the 180 Watt system: a multicenter international study of the of the impact of prostate size on safety and outcomes. J Urol. 2015;194(2):462–9.

38. Mamoulakis C, de La Rosette JMCH. Bipolar transurethral resection of the prostate: Darwinian evolution of an instrumental technique. J Urol. 2015;85(5):1143–50.

39. Giulianelli R, et al. Comparative randomized study on the efficaciousness of treatment of BOO due to BPH in patients with prostate up to 100 gr by endoscopic gyrus prostate resection versus open prostatectomy. Preliminary data. Arch Ital Urol Androl. 2011;83:88–94.

Chapter 12
Robotic Radical Prostatectomy in the Large Prostate

Saskia van der Meer, Veeru Kasivisvanathan, and Ben Challacombe

12.1 Introduction

Over the years global life expectancy has increased. With increasing age prostate size also increases, leaving more and more men at risk of developing prostate cancer in these larger glands. This poses specific problems for cancer treatment, not only for external beam radiotherapy and brachytherapy where very large prostates are often contra-indications, but also for radical surgical treatment. These surgical challenges have been described for the open, laparoscopic (LRP) and robot-assisted technique (RARP) and their different approaches, such as the extraperitoneal or the transperitoneal approach and the anterior or posterior approach. Unfortunately, in the literature, studies with longer follow-up that evaluate the effect of prostate size on operative time, intraoperative complications, oncological and functional outcome, tend to include a mix of all these techniques and approaches. However, these different surgical approaches might have different effects on these outcomes. Furthermore, information about the specific challenges faced with very large prostates exceeding 100 g is scarce.

This chapter will focus on the challenges of robot-assisted laparoscopic radical prostatectomy in these extremely large prostates and hopes to provide some advice on how to overcome them. But first, the possible impact of prostate size on oncological and functional outcome will be discussed.

S. van der Meer (✉)
Erasmus Medical Center, Cancer Institute,
's-Gravendijkwal 230, 3015 CE Rotterdam, The Netherlands
e-mail: s.vandermeer@erasmusmc.nl

V. Kasivisvanathan
University College London and University College London Hospitals,
132 Hampstead Road, London, UK
e-mail: veeru.kasi@ucl.ac.uk

B. Challacombe
MRC Centre for Transplantation, King's College London, Guy's Hospital, London SE1 9RT, UK
e-mail: benchallacombe@doctors.org.uk

© Springer International Publishing AG 2018
V. Kasivisvanathan, B. Challacombe (eds.), *The Big Prostate*,
https://doi.org/10.1007/978-3-319-64704-3_12

12.2   Operative Time, Intra-operative Blood Loss and Length of Hospital Stay

It is thought that large prostates decrease maneuverability, cause impaired visualisation of the surgical field and less appreciation of surgical planes. This could increase operative time, blood loss and ultimately length of hospital stay [1, 2]. In patients undergoing laparoscopic radical prostatectomy it has been shown that operative time is significantly longer with increasing gland volumes [3, 4]. This is also true for robot-assisted radical prostatectomy (RARP). Not only do surgeons in their learning curve require significantly more time to complete a RARP in larger glands, especially in prostates >100 g, mostly attributed to bladder neck reconstruction and anastomosis, but this has also been shown for experienced surgeons with mean operative time reported to be 20 min longer in glands >100 g compared to glands <50 g [5, 6, 7–10]. This increase in operative time can also be explained by the higher incidence of median lobes in larger glands, which in their own right can lengthen operative time and challenge surgical skills and technique [5, 8]. Furthermore, there seems to be an increase in intra-operative blood loss in these larger glands, ranging from an additional 40–145 mL blood loss, with 1.5% needing transfusion, as well as a small increase in other intraoperative complications such as bowel injuries (<1%) with a slightly longer hospital stay as a consequence [6, 7–9]. On the other hand, some authors report no significant increase in operative time, intra-operative blood loss or length of hospital stay in larger prostates, although small study sample size might offer an explanation [1, 11].

12.3   Oncological Outcomes (Table 12.1)

Despite the surgical challenge, increased prostate size seems to have a more favourable outcome after radical prostatectomy compared to smaller glands. An increase in gland size has been reported to correlate with a decreased incidence of high grade prostate cancer at prostatectomy and a lower likelihood of upgrading [6, 7, 12–14]. Men with larger glands are found to be at a lower risk for progression after robot-assisted laparoscopic radical prostatectomy, because they were about 6% less likely to have extracapsular extension (T3 disease) and 3–19% less likely to have positive surgical margins, which was expecially true for men with prostate sizes >100 g [1, 7, 9, 12, 13].

Again, some authors did not find a significant difference in surgical margins or biochemical recurrence related to prostate size [8, 10, 11]. When more positive margins were found in larger prostates this seemed to be due to stage T3 disease [11].

It seems that increased prostate size does not have an adverse effect, but rather seems to be advantageous in terms of oncological outcome.

Table 12.1 Key studies reporting oncological outcomes in patients with large prostates

Study	Number of patients and trial design	Study group	Intervention(s) Length of study	Relevant outcomes
Bishara et al. (2014)	344, Prospective cohort study	Patients undergoing RARP Between 2008 and 2013 In a single centre Prostate size ≥75 g compared to <75 g	RARP 20 months	Prostate size ≥75 g was associated with a lower Gleason score and a lower pathological stage but also with a longer operative time (255 versus 222 min), greater blood loss (349 mL versus 219 mL), and blood transfusion requirements (0.01 versus 0.13 units per operation). Larger prostates (≥75 g) were associated with a longer postoperative stay (2.82 days versus 2.26 days), and longer postoperative catheter time (10.3 days versus 9.2 days). Higher PSA density is independently associated with biochemical recurrence.
Labanaris et al. (2013)	370, Retrospective cohort study	Patients who underwent RARP Between 2006 and 2012 In a single centre Prostate size ≥100 g compared to ≤50 g	RARP 24 months	Prostate size ≥100 g was associated with less aggressive tumors, less positive surgical margins (4.8% versus 10.8%) and a lower incidence of biochemical recurrence. However, they exhibited a significant increase in blood loss (192 mL versus 152 mL), operative time needed (164 min versus 144 min), increased need for bladder neck reconstruction (28.1% versus 5.9%) as well as an increase in intraoperative complications.
Freedland et al. (2005)	1602, Retrospective cohort study (Shared Equal Access Regional Cancer Hospital (SEARCH) Database)	Patients who underwent RP Between 1988 and 2003 In five equal-access medical centers Prostate size increase in 20 g intervals	RP 46 months	Men with smaller prostates had more high-grade cancers, positive surgical margins, extracapsular extension and were at greater risk of progression after RP.

(continued)

Table 12.1 (continued)

Study	Number of patients and trial design	Study group	Intervention(s) Length of study	Relevant outcomes
Hong et al. (2014)	1756, Retrospective cohort study	Patients who underwent preoperative MRI and radical prostatectomy Between 2000 and 2010 In a single centre	Preoperative MRI and RP 5 years	Smaller prostate volume was significantly associated with high pathologic Gleason score, ext racapsular extension, and positive surgical margins. No significant interaction between clinical stage and prostate volume was observed in predicting adverse pathologic features. The association between prostate volume and recurrence was significant in a multivariable analysis adjusting for postoperative variables, but missed statistical significance in the preoperative model.
D'Amico et al. (1998)	885, Prospective cohort study	Patients who underwent RP and bilateral PLND Between 1989 and 1997 Prostate size divided into <30, 30–75 and >75 cm³	RP 42 months	Lead time bias because of PSA driven repeat biopsy accounted for the high 4-year PSA failure free survival and favorable pathologic findings for most patients with a prostate volume in excess of 75 cm³.
Zorn et al. (2007)	375, Prospective cohort study	Patients undergoing RARP Between 2003 and 2005 In a single centre Prostate size divided into <30, 30–50, 50–80 and >80 g	RARP 24 months	No significant differences in operative time, estimated blood loss, transfusion rate, hospital stay, length of catheterization, and complication incidence were observed. Positive surgical margins decreased with larger prostate size, especially in patients with Stage pT2.

Study	N, study type	Description	Procedure, follow-up	Findings
Skolarus et al. (2010)	885, Retrospective cohort study	Patients who underwent RARP. Between 2003 and 2008. In a single centre. Prostate size divided into <50, 50–100, and >100 g	RARP 3 months	Larger prostate size was associated with increased operative times and blood loss, although of questionable clinical significance.
Link et al. (2008)	1847, Prospective cohort study	Patients undergoing RP. Between 2003 and 2007. In a single centre. Prostate size divided into <30, 30–49, 50–69 and ≥70 g	RP (97% RARP) 48 months	Pathologically larger prostates are generally associated with lower Gleason score and risk group stratification. Patients with an enlarged prostate have a slightly longer operative time, higher urinary leakage rates and longer hospital stay.
Huang et al. (2011)	951, Retrospective cohort study	Patients who underwent RARP—Between 2005 and 2010. In a single centre	RARP 24 months	Although BPH characteristics prolonged operative times and increased blood loss, prostate size did not affect positive surgical margins.
Boczko et al. (2007)	355, Prospective cohort study	Patients undergoing RARP. In a single centre. Prostate size <75 g compared to ≥75 g	RARP 6 months	Patients with prostate size ≥75 g had more blood loss (175 mL versus 226 mL). No difference was seen in Gleason score (6 v 6), clinical T stage, operative time (217 min versus 225 min), or total positive-margin rate (13% versus 19%). A higher positive-margin rate was seen in patients with stage T3 disease and larger prostates.

12.4   Functional Outcomes (Table 12.2)

12.4.1   Incontinence

In theory, many factors can influence continence after radical prostatectomy. First, preservation of urethral length is shown to improve continence, therefore resection of a larger part of the urethra during radical prostatectomy due to increased prostate size could influence continence unfavourably in these patients [15]. The access to and intra-operative views of the apex of the prostate are much more difficult in these larger glands.

Also, sparing the bladder neck may better preserve the internal sphincter responsible for passive continence, so the need for a bladder neck reconstruction in large glands may delay or decrease restoration of continence [15, 16].

Another possible impediment on post-prostatectomy continence in men with increased prostate volumes could be the higher incidence of pre-existing LUTS as well as the fact that these men tend to be of older age, making them more likely to exhibit pre-existent bladder and sphincteric dysfunction [9, 15, 16].

Despite the theoretical disadvantages described, the literature is contradictory in the effect of prostate size on regaining continence after radical prostatectomy, whether by laparoscopic approach or by RARP. Some authors describe a prolonged time to restoration of continence for larger glands with 6-month continence rates of 63% in prostates >100 g, but with comparable outcomes to smaller prostates after 1–2 years, while others do not find any significant difference [1 , 7–11, 17].

12.4.2   Erectile Function

One can hypothesise that due to the technical difficulties of operating on a larger prostate, nerve-sparing may also be more of a challenge. However, in some cases men with larger glands have the neurovascular bundles placed very posteriorly in a longitudinal strip making nerve sparing relatively simple once the correct plane is found. The effect of gland size on erectile function is not extensively described in the literature. However, it is described that men with larger prostates have worse baseline sexual function to start with, which could be explained by increasing age [9, 10]. Most studies show that there is no significant difference in regaining baseline erectile function between larger or smaller glands, but recovery in larger prostates does seem to be slower compared to smaller glands, with an 11% lower potency rate at 1 year in larger glands which is recovered with greater time [1, 7, 9, 10].

Table 12.2 Key studies reporting functional outcomes in patients with large prostates

Study	Number of patients and trial design	Main inclusion/exclusion criteria	Intervention(s), length of study	Relevant outcomes
Heesakkers et al. (2016)	Review of 128 studies	Studies on postprostatectomy incontinence Published between 1990 and 2015 In PubMed and Embase	RP 12–24 months	Four studies described postprostatectomy incontinence related to prostate size. One study showed that the 6-month post-RP continence rate was significantly lower for men with prostate size >75 cm³. Another reported that patients with prostate size >50 cm³ had lower rates of continence at 6 and 12 months after RP, but continence rates equalized at 24-months follow-up. However, two other studies revealed that prostate size did not predict post-RP continence outcome, with one study describing that prostate size did not appear to have any effect on functional outcomes.
Ficarra et al. (2012)	Systematic review of 51 studies	Studies on postprostatectomy incontinence Published between 2008 and 2011 In Medline, Embase, and Web of Science	RARP, RP, LRP 12 months	The 12-month urinary incontinence rates ranged from 4% to 31%, with a mean value of 16% using a no pad definition. Considering a no pad or safety pad definition, the incidence ranged from 8% to 11%, with a mean value of 9%. Age, body mass index, comorbidity index, lower urinary tract symptoms, and prostate volume were the most relevant preoperative predictors of urinary incontinence after RARP. Although different values were used in the literature to define a large prostate, a cut-off value between 70 and 80 cm³ could be correlated with a significant risk of urinary incontinence after RARP.

(continued)

Table 12.2 (continued)

Study	Number of patients and trial design	Main inclusion/exclusion criteria	Intervention(s), length of study	Relevant outcomes
Zorn et al. (2007)	375, Prospective cohort study	Patients undergoing RARP Between 2003 and 2005 In a single centre Prostate size divided into <30 g, 30–50 g, 50–80 g and >80 g	RARP 24 months	Return of sexual and urinary function was not affected by prostate size.
Skolarus et al. (2010)	885, Retrospective cohort study	Patients who underwent RARP Between 2003 and 2008 In a single centre Prostate size divided into <50 g, 50–100 g, and >100 g	RARP 3 months	Larger prostate size patients appeared to benefit regarding irritative symptoms, but recovery of continence was delayed.
Labanaris et al. (2013)	370, Retrospective cohort study	Patients who underwent RARP Between 2006 and 2012 In a single centre Prostate size ≥100 g compared to ≤50 g	RARP 24 months	Prostate size ≥100 g was associated with increased need for bladder neck reconstruction, but there was no difference regarding continence rates. However, these large prostates did show significantly lower potency rates (61.9% versus 72.9% potent at 12 months).
Link et al. (2008)	1847, Prospective cohort study	Patients undergoing RP Between 2003 and 2007 In a single centre Prostate size divided into <30 g, 30–49 g, 50–69 g and ≥70 g	RP (97% RARP) 48 months	One-year continence rates are similar across all groups.

Huang et al. (2011)	951, Retrospective cohort study	Patients who underwent RARP Between 2005 and 2010 In a single centre	RARP 24 months	Prostate size did not affect urinary and sexual function.
Boczko et al. (2007)	355, Prospective cohort study	Patients undergoing RARP In a single centre Prostate size <75 g compared to ≥75 g	RARP 6 months	The 6-month continence rate in patients with a prostate volume < 75 g was 97% versus 84% in patients with larger prostate volumes.
Yasui et al. (2014)	219, Retrospective cohort study	Patients who underwent RARP Between 2011 and 2013 In a single centre Prostate size <30 g, 30–49 g, 50–79 g and ≥80 g	RARP 12 months	At 12 months, the urinary continence rates were similar in all groups.

12.5   Other Predictors for a More Challenging RARP

Though increasing prostate size may increase the technical difficulty of a RARP, the role that pelvic cavity dimensions play must also be considered. This remains debatable according to the literature. Hong et al. described that pelvic bone dimensions had no influence on operative time, intra-operative blood loss, surgical margins, recovery of continence or erectile function, and concluded that only gland size had an effect. However, Mason et al. did show that RARP in men with larger prostates and a deep narrow pelvis were more difficult [18, 19]. From our personal experience, we feel that this combination of a deep narrow pelvis and a very large prostate often poses the biggest challenge.

There are different approaches for LRP or RARP, such as the extraperitoneal or the transperitoneal approach and the anterior or posterior approach. There is no one specific superior technique in the literature and all face the same challenges when confronted with large prostates [2, 17]. The transperitoneal approach might provide the surgeon with a little more working space than the extra-peritoneal approach, but the experience and skill of the surgeon will inevitably dictate the outcome.

12.6   Tips and Tricks for RARP in Very Large Prostates
(Table 12.3)

When confronted with a big prostate of more than 100 g it is essential to plan your surgery carefully. It is advisable not to attempt huge glands in your first few cases.

- Always perform an MRI prior to surgery to get a sense of the anatomy and to identify the extremely large prostate.
- There is no evidence to support adjusting the surgical approach to prostate size. Rather, adhere to the approach that one is most accustomed to in order to achieve the best oncological and functional outcome possible.
- Plan trocar placement carefully. Try to optimize the distance between the prostate and the insertion site of the trocars as well as the distance between the individual trocars, in order to improve maneuverability and working space.
- Have good degree of Trendelenberg angulation to improve the pelvic view.
- Clear the working field by fully dropping the bladder, releasing sigmoid and small bowel adhesions, fully dividing the endopelvic fascia to improve the view and surgical exposure.
- Try to preserve as much of the bladder neck as possible to improve continence. A suture through the middle lobe can be used to pull it up towards the abdominal wall in order to improve access to the dorsal part of the bladder neck. If bladder neck preservation is not possible, try to reconstruct it. Take care in tumors at the base of the prostate.

Table 12.3 Key tips and tricks for robot assisted laparoscopic radical prostatectomy in the large prostate

Tips	Rationale
Perform an MRI prior to surgery	Identify the very large prostate prior to surgery to help planning
Pull middle lobe up with a suture	Improve access to the dorsal part of the bladder neck, preserve the bladder neck and improve continence
Anterior bladder suture	Additional exposure of the posterior planes
Cold cutting Santorini complex	Better differentiation between urethral fibers and the prostatic tissue to improve urethal preservation
Rocco stitch	Overcome a large defect after a large-volume prostatectomy and create a tension-free anastomosis
Throw the sutures of the complete dorsal anastomosis before tightening	Improve watertight anastomosis

- Consider a bladder suture on the anterior bladder and clipped through the medial assistant port to give additional exposure of the posterior planes.
- Try to preserve as much of the urethral length as possible. Cold cutting the Santorini complex may provide a better view of the apex, allowing a better differentiation between urethral fibers and the prostatic tissue, though this is not suitable for apical tumors.
- A Rocco stitch may help overcome a large defect after a large-volume prostatectomy by aligning the bladder with the urethra, and can ease tension on the anastomosis.
- Throw the sutures of the complete dorsal anastomosis before tightening. Then carefully pull the sutures to close the dorsal anatomosis, ask the assistant to gently push the bladder towards the anastomosis and then tighten individual throws to secure without tension on the anastomosis.

12.7 Summary

The literature on oncological and functional outcomes after RARP in patients with a prostate size exceeding 100 g is relatively scarce. However, with increasing longevity, the incidence of these extremely large prostates is increasing and it is important to understand how to optimise treatment in these patients.

We know that increased prostate size seems to be advantageous in terms of oncological outcome and that RARP is feasible in these extremely large prostates, but that it poses some challenges.

Our advice is to always perform an MRI when planning surgery, to get a sense of the anatomy and to identify extremely large prostates.

The transperitoneal approach might provide a little more working space than the extra-peritoneal approach, but the experience and skill of the surgeon will dictate the outcome.

During surgery, take care to properly position the patient, optimize trocar placement and clear your surgical field by fully dropping the bladder, releasing sigmoid and small bowel adhesions and fully dividing the endopelvic fascia to improve surgical exposure.

Operative time is described to be slightly longer with large prostates, and blood loss can be slightly more, but although this is statistically significant in some studies, it seems not to be clinically relevant.

For optimal functional outcomes, spare the bladder neck as much as possible or take the time to reconstruct it. A suture through the middle lobe can improve access to the dorsal part of the bladder neck and consider a bladder suture on the anterior bladder to provide additional exposure of the posterior planes. Spare as much of the urethral length as oncologically possible by cold cutting the dorsal venous complex to allow a better view of the apex of the prostate. Consider a Rocco stich for a tension-free anastomosis and throw the sutures of the complete dorsal anastomosis before tightening.

Men with larger prostates seem to have worse baseline sexual function to start with, and recovery after nerve-sparing surgery can be slower, but this seems not to be significantly different. In larger glands nerve sparing can sometimes be easier than in smaller glands because the neurovascular bundles tend to be placed more posteriorly in a longitudinal strip.

References

1. Zorn KC, Orvieto MA, Mikhail AA, et al. Effect of prostate weight on operative and postoperative outcomes of robotic-assisted laparoscopic prostatectomy. Urology. 2007;69:300–5.
2. Santok GD, Abdel Raheem A, Kim LH, Chang K, Lum TG, Chung BH, Choi YD, Rha KH. Perioperative and short-term outcomes of Retzius-sparing robot-assisted laparoscopic radical prostatectomy stratified by gland size. BJU Int. 2016; doi:10.1111/bju.13632.
3. Chang CM, Moon D, Gianduzzo TR, et al. The impact of prostate size in laparoscopic radical prostatectomy. Eur Urol. 2005:285–90.
4. El-Feel A, Davis JW, Deger S, et al. Laparoscopic radical prostatectomy-an analysis of factors affecting operating time. Urology. 2003:314–8.
5. Martinez C, Chalasani V, Lim D, et al. Effect of prostate gland size on the learning curve for robot-assisted laparoscopic radical prostatectomy: does size matter? J Endourol. 2010:261–6.
6. Bishara S, Vasdev N, Lane T, Boustead G, Adshead J. Robotic Prostatectomy has a superior outcome in larger prostates and PSA density is a strong predictor of biochemical recurrence. Prostate Cancer. 2014;763863
7. Labanaris AP, Zugor V, Witt JH. Robot-assisted radical prostatectomy in patients with a pathologic prostate specimen weight ≥100 grams versus ≤50 grams: surgical, oncologic and short-term functional outcomes. Urol Int. 2013:24–30.
8. Link B, Nelson R, Josephson D, et al. The impact of prostate gland weight in robot assisted laparoscopic radical prostatectomy. J Urol. 2008;180:928–32.

9. Skolarus TA, Hedgepeth RC, Zhang Y, Weizer AZ, Montgomery JS, Miller DC, Wood DP Jr, Hollenbeck BK. Does robotic technology mitigate the challenges of large prostate size? Urology. 2010;76:1117–21.
10. Huang AC, Kowalczyk KJ, Hevelone ND, et al. The impact of prostate size, median lobe, and prior benign prostatic hyperplasia intervention on robot-assisted laparoscopic prostatectomy: technique and outcomes. Eur Urol. 2011;59:595–603.
11. Boczko J, Erturk E, Golijanin D, Madeb R, Patel H, Joseph JV. Impact of prostate size in robot-assisted radical prostatectomy. J Endourol. 2007:184–8.
12. Freedland SJ, Isaacs WB, Platz EA, Terris MK, Aronson WJ, Amling CL, et al. Prostate size and risk of high-grade, advanced prostate cancer and biochemical progression after radical prostatectomy: a search database study. J Clin Oncol. 2005:7546–54.
13. Hong SK, Poon BY, Sjoberg DD, Scardino PT, Eastham JA. Prostate size and adverse pathologic features in men undergoing radical prostatectomy. Urology. 2014;84:153–7.
14. D'Amico AV, Whittington R, Malkowicz SB, et al. A prostate gland volume of more than 75 cm^3 predicts for a favorable outcome after radical prostatectomy for localized prostate cancer. Urology. 1998;52:631–6.
15. Heesakkers J, Farag F, Bauer RM, Sandhu J, De Ridder D, Stenzl A. Pathophysiology and contributing factors in postprostatectomy incontinence: a review. Eur Urol. 2016. pii: S0302-2838(16)30666-2.
16. Ficarra V, Novara G, Rosen RC, Artibani W, Carroll PR, Costello A, Menon M, Montorsi F, Patel VR, Stolzenburg JU, Van der Poel H, Wilson TG, Zattoni F, Mottrie A. Systematic review and meta-analysis of studies reporting urinary continence recovery after robot-assisted radical prostatectomy. Eur Urol. 2012;62:405–17.
17. Yasui T, Tozawa K, Kurokawa S, et al. Impact of prostate weight on perioperative outcomes of robot-assisted laparoscopic prostatectomy with a posterior approach to the seminal vesicle. BMC Urol. 2014;14:6.
18. Hong SK, Lee ST, Kim SS, Min KE, Hwang IS, Kim M, Jeong SJ, Byun SS, Hwang SI, Lee SE. Effect of bony pelvic dimensions measured by preoperative magnetic resonance imaging on performing robot-assisted laparoscopic prostatectomy. BJU Int. 2009;104:664–8.
19. Mason BM, Hakimi AA, Faleck D, Chernyak V, Rozenblitt A, Ghavamian R. The role of preoperative endo-rectal coil magnetic resonance imaging in predicting surgical difficulty for robotic prostatectomy. Urology. 2010;76:1130–5.

Chapter 13
Special Conditions: Management of Concomitant Urological Pathology and the Comorbid Patient

Jonathan Makanjuola and Matthew Bultitude

13.1 Endoscopic Management of Concomitant Urological Pathology in Men with >100 cc Prostate

The enlarged prostate (>100 cc) can cause challenges for the most experienced of endourologists. Bleeding from an enlarged gland before the procedure has begun can mean abandoning the procedure, diathermy to stop bleeding and inserting a three-way catheter with continuous bladder irrigation. The ureteric orifices can be very tricky to locate especially if the enlarged gland has middle lobe and/or in bladders with significant trabeculation and diverticula. They can be tucked behind the middle lobe making cannulation with a guide wire problematic and lengthening the operative time. Issues regarding to the surgery can be anticipated by looking at the CT scan pre operatively to assess prostate size.

13.1.1 Rigid and Flexible Ureteroscopy

Most endourologists can usually overcome the challenges of the larger prostate. However, on occasion the very enlarged prostate, particularly with a significant middle lobe, can distort the bladder anatomy making the ureteric orifices difficult or almost impossible to locate. We propose a few tips and tricks for ureteroscopy in the presence of a very large prostate from our personal experience (Table 13.1):

J. Makanjuola, BSc (Hons), AKC, FRCS (Urol.) (✉) • M. Bultitude, M.Sc., F.R.C.S. (Urol.)
The Stone Unit, Department of Urology, Guy's and St Thomas' NHS Foundation Trust,
Great Maze Pond, London SE1 9RT, UK
e-mail: jonathan.makanjuola@nhs.net; matthew.bultitude@gmail.com

© Springer International Publishing AG 2018   167
V. Kasivisvanathan, B. Challacombe (eds.), *The Big Prostate*,
https://doi.org/10.1007/978-3-319-64704-3_13

Table 13.1 A summary of the key tips and tricks for ureteroscopy in the presence of a very large prostate

• Don't make the prostate bleed before you've seen the ureteric orifice
• Preload a hydrophilic tipped wire in a ureteric catheter with the cystoscope
• Look for the contralateral ureteric orifice
• Use an angled hydrophilic guide wire
• Safety wires and stronger wires
• Percutaneous antegrade ureteroscopy
• Planning is key
• Ureteric access sheath
• Post-operative stenting
• Post-operative catheter

- Don't make the prostate bleed before you've seen the ureteric orifice. A bleeding prostate provides additional challenges to the endourologist. This will have to be dealt with before proceeding. In rare circumstances a limited resection of the obstructing middle or lateral lobes of the prostate and diathermy has to be performed. This is likely to need prior consent if one is aware of the potential issue or further consent at a re-operation. On some occasions, if clear vision is impaired, the procedure will have to be abandoned and an irrigating catheter inserted.

- Preload a hydrophilic tipped wire in a ureteric catheter with the cystoscope. The first view will be the best view. Have the right wire ready to insert into the ureteric orifice once it comes into view. Having to change wires could lose the view and can be a struggle to find it again especially if there is then contact bleeding on the prostate. As always, ensure the bladder is empty before ureteroscopy once the guidewire is successfully placed in the renal pelvis.

- Look for the contralateral ureteric orifice. If the ipsilateral ureteric orifice cannot be identified, check for the contralateral one. The intra-ureteric bar is often a good reference point and you may find the orifice is more lateral than you realised. Following the bar laterally should get you to the ureteric orifice on either side.

- Use an angled hydrophilic guide wire. The "fish-hook" configuration of the distal ureter in huge prostates can be difficult to cannulate. The "fish-hook" shape of the distal ureter can be an indirect sign of prostate obstruction and might be caused by a prostate median lobe elevating the trigone. This can displace the ureteral orifices, and deform the distal ureter [3].

- Safety wires and stronger wires. Safety wires should always be used to reduce the risk of loss of the working wire (some would say this is true for all ureteroscopy). Sometimes we have found it helpful to exchange the wire for a stronger wire (e.g. Super Stiff™) to maintain access and help scope passage.

- Percutaneous antegrade ureteroscopy. The European Urology Association (EAU), suggests percutaneous antegrade removal of ureteral stones is a consideration in selected cases or when the ureter is not amenable to retrograde manipulation [1]. This is certainly an option where endoscopic access through the bladder isn't possible.

- Planning is key. If known pre-operatively that the prostate is potentially large and difficult, ensure that the patient is appropriately counselled about the options of antregrade approach or prostatic resection if deemed appropriate under the same anaesthetic. An alternative is arranging for an antegrade stent insertion prior to the surgery. This will help identify the ureteric orifice and also dilate the ureter making manipulation within the ureter easier.

- Ureteric access sheath. Due to the angle over the prostate to the ureteric orifice an access sheath may be required to allow passage of a flexible ureterosope (as it buckles away when trying to pass it over the prostate otherwise). The use of the ureteric access sheath will facilitate the use of the flexible ureteroscope when multiple passes are anticipated, thus reducing contact bleeding from the prostate.

- Post-operative stenting. It is very likely you will want to leave a stent given difficulty of placing one later if needed. Always consider how long this is required for. The stent is likely to make pre-existing lower urinary tract symptoms worse. It may also be challenging to remove under local anaesthesia. A tether left on the stent will avoid this problem if only needed for a short period of time. The use of a Polaris™ Loop Ureteral Stent (Boston Scientific) may reduce bladder irritation and contact bleeding.

- Post-operative catheter. The patient undergoing an endoscopic procedure with a huge 100 cc prostate will be at high risk of post-operative retention and a catheter should be placed at the end of the operation. It is useful to know whether a standard catheter can be passed without the use of a guidewire or introducer in case of future need for catheterisation. In the pre-operative consent process the potential for urinary retention and the need for a bladder outflow procedure should be highlighted.

13.1.2 Transurethral Resection of a Bladder Tumour (TURBT)

A transurethral resection of a bladder tumour (TURBT) is one of the most common operations in urology [2]. Problems can be encountered before the resection of the bladder tumour has begun in men with a huge prostate. At the start of the operation a large prostate can cause prostatic bleeding obscuring the view of the bladder tumour. This can limit identification of the primary tumour or other smaller lesions including the red patch associated with carcinoma in situ particularly if the tumour is hidden behind an obstructing middle lobe. A transurethral resection of the prostate (TURP) may have to be performed before the TURBT (with appropriate consent). If the prostate gland is causing bleeding that is obstructing the view of the bladder limiting safe bladder resection it would be appropriate to resect and diathermy the prostate. Creation of a channel in the prostate is the most appropriate if there is no history of LUTS and the main goal is not improving flow. If there is a middle lobe of the prostate gland limiting visualisation of the bladder tumour resection of the middle lobe is appropriate to gain better views of the tumour. Use of extra long resectoscopes can be used if no bleeding is present but the enlarged prostate makes it difficult to get the bladder mass to resect. Benign prostatic enlargement (BPE) is most commonly encountered in elderly men, with the incidence rising with the ageing population [3]. It is not unusual to encounter the clinical scenario of a male patient undergoing endoscopic treatment for bladder tumour with a TURBT that may also require concurrent TURP. It was previously unclear whether it was safe to combine the two procedures since there was a theoretical risk of circulating cancer cells that may implant into the raw prostatic fossa and thereby enhance the risk of subsequent recurrences in the prostatic fossa [4]. This is now thought to be safe to do [5] following a meta-analysis of six eligible clinical trials looking at 483 patients treated with simultaneous prostate resection and TURBT vs. 500 with TURBT alone. Within the follow-up periods there was no difference in tumour recurrence between the groups including recurrence in the prostatic fossa. Overall the combined analysis actually indicated lower recurrence rates in the simultaneous resection group in the overall (combined OR = 0.67; 95% CI 0.52–0.88, P = 0.003). A catheter will be required post-operatively and it is useful to decide whether the patient can be catheterised normally, especially as the patient may require future catheterisation for intravesical mitomycin or BCG. This is also relevant as if the prostate bleeds easily with catheterisation then proceeding with the intravesical instillation may be contraindicated.

In the presence of multiple bladder tumours starting resections anteriorly/at the dome of the bladder may be preferable, leaving tumours which are located in a region that requires manipulation of an enlarged prostate lobe until later, to reduce contact bleeding. This will ensure the view is adequate for resection around the bladder dome.

Anaesthetic considerations in TURBT of tumours in the vicinity of the obturator nerve. It is essential that muscle relaxation is given. In a large bladder tumour in addition to a large obstructive prostate this may cause increased bleeding and increase the difficulty of the procedure by poor visualisation of the bladder.

13.1.3   Cystolitholapaxy (Bladder Stone Removal)

Surgical treatment is usually required when patients have bladder stones [6] as the chance of recurrence is high if bladder outflow surgery isn't performed simultaneously. When performing transurethral cystolitholapaxy a good view is critical to prevent inadvertent bladder injury with the sharp jaws of the Mauermayer punch. The large prostate may well prevent access to the stone over the bladder neck. It is likely that most men presenting with bladder stones will need dis-obstruction with either separate or concomitant bladder outflow surgery.

If planning on preforming a cystolitholapaxy but cannot quite sufficiently get hold of the stone due to a large prostate, one strategy would be to preform a TURP to gain a channel in the prostate and then finish with cystolitholapaxy. Alternatively it might be the case that a TURP and cystolitholapaxy is planned in a man with known bladder stones. The TURP should be preformed first to ensure there is less risk of bleeding from the enlarged prostate. Poor visualisation during cystolitholapaxy due to bleeding from the enlarge prostate increasing the chances of intraoperative complication such as iatrogenic bladder injury.

In men who have a large prostate gland, holmium laser cystolitholapaxy can be safely combined with holmium laser enucleation of the prostate (HoLEP) [7]. This avoids use of the stone punch and may thus reduce the incidence of bladder mucosal injury. Sometimes larger burden bladder stones (>2 cm diameter) may require a percutaneous or an open procedure. These approaches may not be feasible in certain patients who are at increased risk of operative complications and bleeding.

13.1.4 Upper Urinary Tract Procedures

Men requiring a partial nephrectomy, pyeloplasty, percutaneous nephrolithotomy, or open stone surgery who have concomitant significant bladder outflow obstruction are at risk of complications due to the large prostate causing increased upper tract pressures. In the case of laparoscopic procedures a urinary leak at the anastomosis or rennorraphy site is possible whilst in PCLN or open kidney surgery a urinary fistula to the skin can develop with subqeuent sequelae of infection and delayed discharge likely. To avoid this the lower urinary tract should be fully disobstructed first, prior to the upper tract procedure.

13.2 Management of Co-morbid, Frail or Elderly Men with Prostates >100 cc

13.2.1 Patient Selection

Older people undergoing elective surgery have increased risk of significant postoperative problems prolonging hospitalisation, increasing morbidity and mortality [8]. Ageing is associated with independent risk factors for adverse postoperative and post-oncological outcomes [9]. These risk factors can be categorised as (1) physiological decline with a consequent reduction in functional reserve, (2) comorbidities and (3) geriatric syndromes, such as frailty. To reduce the impact of these risk factors on postoperative morbidity and mortality, it is essential that this high-risk population undergo individualised assessment, optimisation and medical management [10]. Recent data indicate that frailty is a more powerful predictor of increased perioperative mortality and morbidity than predictions based on age or comorbidity alone [11, 12]. Frail surgical patients are less likely to be discharged to home [13], more likely to be readmitted to the hospital within 30 days [14] and more likely to have increased rates of postoperative complications [14].

When considering surgical options for elderly men with big prostates, assessment of prostate volume is even more important than usual for the selection of appropriate interventional treatment in men with lower urinary tract symptoms (LUTS) [15]. Accurate calculation of prostate volume also predicts symptom progression, risk of retention, and the risk of complications in older man undergoing bladder outflow surgery [15]. Uroflowmetry and International Prostate Symptom Score (IPSS) questionnaires [16] should be used in combination to determine men who need bladder outflow surgery.

Uroflowmetry might not be easy to obtain in older patients, as voiding on demand can be problematic and they commonly void small volumes and may have associated urgency or urgency incontinence [16]. Preoperative urodynamic tests are advised for accurate clinical diagnosis in the older co-morbid man with LUTS when there is difficulty in establishing the underlying diagnosis (e.g. elderly men with Parkinson's disease or other neurological diseases) [17]. In men with voiding LUTS, benign prostate enlargement (BPE) with ageing causes benign prostatic obstruction (BPO) [18]. For such patients, prostate surgery, has a good chance of improving LUTS [18]. Voiding LUTS can also be caused by bladder dysfunction this is often referred to as 'the underactive bladder' [19]. In such men, it is hard to justify prostate surgery if BPO is not present, especially in view of potential adverse effects associated with surgery, such as blood transfusion requirement, problems of sexual function, anaesthetic problems or incontinence [18].

13.2.2 Medical Optimisation

There are emerging new models of care for older surgical patients such as Proactive care for Older Patients undergoing Surgery (POPS) [8]. Indicators like the Charlson comorbidity index, Frailty Screening [20, 21] or Cardio Pulmonary Exercise Testing (CPET) [22] predict postoperative morbidity and mortality. The POPS service is designed to predict postoperative morbidity and mortality for patients who may have a range of co-morbidities. Preoperative comprehensive geriatric assessment can identify elderly patients at greater risk for mortality, post-discharge institutionalisation, adverse in-hospital events, and prolonged length of hospital stay [23]. We recommend all frail elderly patients are seen pre-operatively by care of the elderly physicians and anaesthetists as part of the preoperative assessment. Cardiovascular status needs to be determined with electrocardiogram (ECG) and often left ventricular function via echocardiography (echo). Post operative risk assessment of delirium by medication review and identifying strategies to minimise the effects. At this time a haematology consult can ensure a pre and post operative plan can be documented regarding anti- coagulation stop and start dates.

This is in addition to assessment, optimisation and management of complex older surgical patients is required. At times medications can have a role in pre-treatment in men with LUTS to improve the surgical outcomes in men with big prostates. Pre-treatment with 5 alpha reductase inhibitors has been shown in a number of studies to reduce perioperative blood loss related to TURP for BPH patients [24]. This effect is probably due to decreased vascularity in the prostate rather than a smaller prostate volume or shorter operative time [24].

13.2.3 Choice of Anaesthesia

Once the patient has been pre-assessed and medically optimised there are still intra operative challenges that face the anaesthetist in the elderly, frail and co-morbid patients. The choice of anaesthesia can have an impact on morbidity. Elderly patients are at risk for postoperative delirium. Drugs used in anaesthesia (such as benzodiaz-epines and anticholinergic drugs) are known to precipitate or exacerbate postopera-tive delirium in older patients [25]. Selective spinal anaesthesia is an alternative to general anaesthesia and provides appropriate sensory block for TURP in elderly patients [26]. The major problem with the spinal technique is risk of hypotension. As a result of the spinal induced sympathetic blockade, there is vasodilatation lead-ing to diminished venous return, which is the main contributory factor for hypoten-sion [27]. In elderly patients with cardiac disease systemic vascular resistance may decrease. This hypotension is usually corrected by either administration of intrave-nous (i.v.) fluids or vasopressor. Liberal use of i.v. fluid administration is dangerous particularly elderly patients with compromised cardiopulmonary function [28]. The elderly are more sensitive to anaesthetics, meaning that desired sedative and analge-sic effects are reached at lower doses compared with younger patients, and the hae-modynamic depressing side effects of anaesthetics are often more pronounced [28].

13.2.4 Post-operative Management

Post-operatively it has been show by studies that elderly patients have better out-comes if the care-of-the-elderly physicians are proactively reviewing the patients daily and working with the surgical teams [29–31]. Medical and social care within a multidisciplinary team (MDT) structure for preoperative optimisation, and post-operative management by highlighting geriatric issues on the ward, showed improved rates for discharge directly home in elective and emergency surgical patients [30]. Delirium is an important complication in the elderly because it results in functional decline, longer hospitalisation, and institutionalisation [31]. Delirium-specific complications include falls, pulled lines/tubes, aspiration pneumonia, and increased use of bladder catheters [32]. Patients who develop delirium during their hospitalisation have a higher 6-month mortality in comparison with patients who do not develop delirium [33–37].

13.3 Conclusion

The enlarged prostate (>100 cc) can cause challenges for the most experienced of endourologists. Problems arising from the big prostate in common endourological procedures can be overcome with correct planning and operative maneuverers. This chapter highlights the importance of patient selection, identification of high-risk groups and how medical optimisation pre-operatively can improve outcomes in elderly men with large prostates undergoing endourological procedures. Patient factors have been shown to be stronger predictors of mortality than the type of surgery undertaken. Multidisciplinary co-ordination with care of the elderly physicians, surgeons and anaesthetists pre operatively can optimise the elderly and comorbid man with the big prostate.

References

1. Brodak M, Tomasek J, Pacovsky J, Holub L, Husek P. Urological surgery in elderly patients: results and complications. Clin Interv Aging. 2015;10:379–85. doi:10.2147/CIA.S73381.
2. Story DA, Leslie K, Myles PS, et al. Complications and mortality in older surgical patients in Australia and New Zealand (the REASON study): a multicentre, prospective, observational study. Anaesthesia. 2010;65(10):1022–30. doi:10.1111/j.1365-2044.2010.06478.
3. Mamoulakis C, Herrmann TRW, Höfner K, et al. The fish-hook configuration of the distal ureter indicates bladder outlet obstruction due to benign prostatic hyperplasia. World J Urol. 2011;29(2):199–204. doi:10.1007/s00345-010-0612-9.
4. Türk C, Petřík A, Sarica K, et al EAU guidelines on interventional treatment for urolithiasis. Eur Urol. 2016;69(3):475–82. doi: 10.1016.
5. Lee F, Patel HR, Emberton M. The 'top 10' urological procedures: a study of hospital episodes statistics 1998–99. BJU Int. 2002;90:1–6.
6. Rowhrborm CG, McConnell JD. Etiology, pathophysiology, epidemiology and natural history of benign prostatic hyperplasia. In: Walsh PC, Retik AB, Vaughan Jr ED, Wein AJ, editors. Campbell's urology. Philadelphia: W. B. Saunders; 2002. p. 1297–330.
7. Li S, Zeng X-T, Raun XL, et al. Simultaneous transurethral resection of bladder cancer and prostate may reduce recurrence rates: A systematic review and meta-analysis. Exp Ther Med. 2012;4(4):685–92. Epub 2012 Aug 9
8. Luo S, Lin Y, Zhang W. Does simultaneous transurethral resection of bladder tumor and prostate affect the recurrence of bladder tumor? A meta-analysis J Endourol. 2011;25(2):291–6. doi:10.1089/end.2010.0314. Epub 2010 Oct 26
9. Gratzke C, Bachmann A, Descazeaud A, et al. EAU Guidelines on the Assessment of Non-neurogenic Male Lower Urinary Tract Symptoms including Benign Prostatic Obstruction. Eur Urol. 2015;67(6):1099–109. doi:10.1016/j.eururo.2014.12.038. Epub 2015 Jan 19
10. Tangpaitoon T, Marien T, Kadihasanoglu M et al. Does cystitholapaxy at the time of holmium laser enucleation of the prostate affect outcomes? Urology. 2017;99:192–196.

11. Harari D, Hopper A, Dhesi J, et al. Proactive care of older people undergoing surgery ('POPS'): designing, embedding, evaluating and funding a comprehensive geriatric assessment service for older elective surgical patients. Age Ageing. 2007;36:190–6.
12. Abu-Ghanem Y, Dhesi JK, Challacombe BJ. The challenges of managing urological malignancy in the elderly. BJU Int. 2014;114(1):12–5. doi:10.1111/bju.12617.
13. Turrentine FE, Wang H, Simpson VB, et al. Surgical risk factors, morbidity, and mortality in elderly patients. J Am Coll Surg. 2006;203(6):865–77.
14. Robinson TN, Wu DS, Pointer L, et al. Simple frailty score predicts postoperative complications across surgical specialties. Am J Surg. 2013;206(4):544–50.
15. Makary MA, Segev DL, Pronovost PJ, et al. Frailty as a predictor of surgical outcomes in older patients. J Am Coll Surg. 2010;210(6):901–8.
16. McAdams-DeMarco MA, Law A, Salter ML, et al. Frailty and early hospital readmission after kidney transplantation. Am J Transplant. 2013;13(8):2091–5.
17. Hall DE, Arya S, Schmid KK, et al. Association of a Frailty Screening Initiative with postoperative survival at 30, 180, and 365 days. JAMA Surg. 2016; doi:10.1001/jamasurg.2016.4219.
18. Wilkinson AG, Wild SR. Is pre-operative imaging of the urinary tract worthwhile in the assessment of prostatism? Br J Urol. 1992;70:53.
19. Cockett ATK, Aso Y, Denis L, et al. World Health Organization Consensus Committee recommendations concerning the diagnosis of BPH. Prog Urol. 1991;1(6):957–72.
20. Abdul-Rahman A, Al-Hayek S, Belal M. Urodynamic studies in the evaluation of the older man with lower urinary tract symptoms: when, which ones, and what to do with the results. Ther Adv Urol. 2010;2(5–6):187–94. doi:10.1177/1756287210385924.
21. Bailey K, Abrams P, Blair PS, et al. Urodynamics for Prostate Surgery Trial; Randomised Evaluation of Assessment Methods (UPSTREAM) for diagnosis and management of bladder outlet obstruction in men: study protocol for a randomised controlled trial. Trials. 2015;16:567. doi:10.1186/s13063-015-1087-1.
22. Osman N, Mangera A, Hillary C et al. The underactive bladder: detection and diagnosis. F1000Research. 2016;5:F1000 Faculty Rev-102. doi:10.12688/f1000research.7344.1.
23. Fried LP, Tangen CM, Walston J, et al. Frailty in older adults: evidence for a phenotype. J Gerontol A Biol Sci Med Sci. 2001;56:M146–56.
24. Bandeen-Roche K, Xue QL, Ferrucci L, et al. Phenotype of frailty: characterization in the women's health and aging studies. J Gerontol A Biol Sci Med Sci. 2006;61:262–6.
25. MacGregor T, Patel N, Blick C, et al. Is there a role for cardiopulmonary exercise testing before major urological surgery. BJU Int. 2009;104(5):579–80. doi:10.1111/j.1464-410X.2009.08517.x. Epub 2009 Apr 17
26. Kim KI, Park KH, Koo KH, et al. Comprehensive geriatric assessment can predict post operative morbidity and mortality in elderly patients undergoing elective surgery. Arch Gerontol Geriatr. 2013;56(3):507–12. doi:10.1016/j.archger.2012.09.002. Epub 2012 Dec 14
27. Zhu YP, Dai B, Zhang HL. Impact of preoperative 5α-reductase inhibitors on perioperative blood loss in patients with benign prostatic hyperplasia: a meta-analysis of randomized controlled trials. BMC Urol. 2015;15:47. doi:10.1186/s12894-015-0043-4.
28. Tomlinson JH, Partridge JSL. Preoperative discussion with patients about delirium risk: are we doing enough? Perioperative Medicine. 2016;5(1):22. doi:10.1186/s13741-016-0047-y.
29. Kim NY, Kim SY. Ju HM, et al Selective Spinal Anesthesia Using 1 mg of Bupivacaine with Opioid in Elderly Patients for Transurethral Resection of Prostate. Yonsei Med J. 2015;56(2):535–42. doi:10.3349/ymj.2015.56.2.535.
30. Bhattacharyya S, Bisai S, Biswas H, et al. Regional anesthesia in transurethral resection of prostate (TURP) surgery: A comparative study between saddle block and subarachnoid block. Saudi J Anaesth. 2015;9(3):268–71. doi:10.4103/1658-354X.158497.
31. Strøm C, Rasmussen LS, Steinmetz J. Practical management of anaesthesia in the elderly. Drugs Aging. 2016;33(11):765–77.
32. Braude, P., Goodman, A., Elias, T., et al. Evaluation and establishment of a ward-based geriatric liaison service for older urological surgical patients: Proactive care of Older People undergoing Surgery (POPS)-Urology. BJU Int. 2016;120(1):123-129. doi:10.1111/bju.13526.

33. Partridge JSL, Harari D, Dhesi JK. Frailty in the older surgical patient: a review. Age Ageing. 2012;41:142–7.
34. Patel SA, Zenilman ME. Outcomes in older people undergoing operative intervention for colorectal cancer. J Am Geriatr Soc. 2001;49:1561–4.
35. Robinson TN, Eiseman B. Postoperative delirium in the elderly: diagnosis and management. Clin Interv Aging. 2008;3(2):351–5.
36. Demeure MJ, Fain MJ. The elderly surgical patient and postoperative delirium. J Am Coll Surg. 2006;203:752–7.
37. Ely EW, Shintani A, Truman B, et al. Delirium as a predictor of mortality in mechanically ventilated patients in the intensive care unit. JAMA. 2004;291:1753–62.

Chapter 14
The Future of Management of Benign Prostatic Hyperplasia

Gideon Adam Blecher, Rick Leslie Catterwell, and Ben Challacombe

14.1 Introduction

Before we can predict what the future holds for treatment of benign prostate hyperplasia (BPH), we must understand its past. John Hunter described prostatic enlargement and the development of an obstructing middle lobe with bladder trabeculation in the 1786 and even elucidated the relationship between the testes and prostatic growth. In 1830, Englishman George Gurthrie described insertion of a blade to incise an obstruction. Forty-four years later, Italian Enrico Bottini introduced electrical current, although this instrument was blind until American Maximilian Stern performed a transurethral resection of prostate (TURP) in 1926 with a visual resectoscope. These steps were clearly a major advancement, enabling minimally invasive treatment. Despite utilisation of glycine at this stage, further improvements in technology and technique, anaesthetic and surgical risks have developed. A variety of surgical energy sources and approaches have flourished, including holmium laser enucleation. Again, these are not complication free.

Emerging medical treatments via the introduction of alpha-blockers was likely the next major step in BPH management. Since then, further medical therapies have arrived including selective alpha blockers (ABs), five-alpha-reductase inhibitors (5ARIs) and phosphodiesterase-5-inhibitor (PDE5Is). More recently the combination of these drugs have become commonplace. Although these medications

G.A. Blecher (✉) • R.L. Catterwell
Guy's and St Thomas' NHS Trust, London, UK
e-mail: docblecher@gmail.com; rick.catterwell@gmail.com

B. Challacombe
Guy's and St Thomas' NHS Trust, London, UK

King's College London, London, UK
e-mail: benchallacombe@doctors.org.uk

© Springer International Publishing AG 2018
V. Kasivisvanathan, B. Challacombe (eds.), *The Big Prostate*,
https://doi.org/10.1007/978-3-319-64704-3_14

improve the situation with regards to symptoms, 'perfect flow rates' or unanimous International Prostate Symptom Scores of zero, are rarely achieved. Adverse effects including postural hypotension, retrograde ejaculation, erectile dysfunction and reduced libido are just some of the problems patients experience whilst on such treatments. The long-term patient/community cost of such medicines is also significant.

Prostatic artery embolization (PAE) is an emerging minimally invasive option. It is likely to have a role in the niche after medications but prior to surgery, however, more long-term data would be desirable.

Not only has BPH specific technology in this area changed, but the future patient will not necessarily be the same as today. World-wide life expectancies are increasing [1], as such, BPH patients will be older, frailer and more medically comorbid. As the range of various treatment options expand, patients will utilise multiple lines of treatment, such that the men who fail first line medical treatments, may have larger glands by the time it comes to second, third, fourth or later lines of management. Previously a prostate over 100 cc in size was a rarity but with increasing numbers of men undergoing long term medical treatments for BPH, prostates over 250 cc in size are now not uncommon.

So what are we aiming for in terms of the optimal potential treatment? Ideally, in the future, we will have access to a magic bullet; a treatment which can manage all varieties of prostate size, have minimal risks and minimal adverse effects. It should be readily accessible and deliverable to all corners of the world, whilst being efficient and inexpensive. A lack of, or minimal learning curve and long-term durability are similarly desirable. There are clearly many roadblocks to such a treatment, but as new technologies arise, these are the qualities we should be demanding.

14.2   Medical Treatments

Utilisation rates for alpha-blockers have increased over the past few decades. From 1993 until 2010, US rates of alpha-blocker prescriptions for BPH/LUTS rose from 14 to 40% [2]. Similar patterns have been demonstrated in Italy and Iceland [3, 4]. It is predicted that a medical treatment may ultimately fulfill many of the criteria of the ideal treatment and there are multiple experimental drugs that will be briefly discussed.

Alpha-blockers have varying degrees of alpha-1 receptor selectivity, which alters their side effect profile. There may exist other determinants of their adverse effects. Although there is a paucity of head to head trials, it is likely that they exhibit similar effectiveness [5]. There exist several subtypes of alpha-1 receptor (α1a-AR, α1b-AR, α1d-AR): undoubtedly these will be further explored. It is suggested that genetic background variation in patients with BPH, will enable more personalized utilization of such subtypes, whilst genetic profiling studies may enable an additional method of assessing response [6].

Not only will newer agents with a more personalized genetic based approach be developed, but new combinations of drugs will demonstrate cumulative effects. Landmark studies such as MTOPS [7] and ComBAT [8] provide evidence supporting guideline recommendations of combination 5-alpha-reductase inhibitor plus alpha-blocker for the treatment of moderate to severe lower urinary tract symptoms (LUTS). Combination PDE5I and AB or 5ARI, or antimuscurinics plus AB are further examples. It is likely that pharmaceutical research will unveil new combination treatments, which demonstrate higher efficacy and better tolerability than current options. Despite the advantage of such combinations, it should be considered that polypharmacy, particularly in a likely older and more comorbid population, may have its disadvantages.

14.3 Experimental Medical Treatments

A variety of experimental drugs are noted in the literature, however robust long term controlled trial data is not yet available.

NX-1207 is an experimental compound with selective pro-apoptotic properties, which is administered via intraprostatic injection. Animal studies show a reduction in prostate volume of 40–47% over twelve months. Human trials demonstrate a 90-day reduction in AUA Symptom Score of 9.7 compared to 4.7 with finasteride [9]. Preclinical animal and phase III human trials have not demonstrated any significant toxicity or safety concerns.

PRX302 is an inactive modified form of bacterial cytolytic protein, which is also directly injected into the adenoma. Prostate specific antigen (PSA) is involved in its activation [10]. In a phase II trial, 61% of patients at one year demonstrated a >3 mL/s improvement in flow rate. No change in flow was noted in the phase I trial. Prostate volume was decreased by >20% in 87% of patients at 90 days, and by 27% at 1 year [11].

Elocalcitol is a Vitamin D3 receptor (VDR) analogue, which aims to inhibit cell reproduction and also induces prostatic cellular apoptosis [12] via interleukin-8 dependent pathways [13]. A randomized human trial in human BPH patients demonstrated a −7.22% difference (95% confidence interval −9.27 to −5.18, $p < 0.0001$) in prostate volume change at 12 weeks compared to placebo, and though there were not any significant effect on flow rates [14], the prostate size reduction showed good promise for future work.

Exploiting BPHs reliance on androgens, there have been several studies looking into the role of gonadotrophin-releasing-hormone antagonists. Teverelix has shown a reduction in International Prostate Symptom Score (IPSS) of 6.3 at 16 weeks, as well as 11.5% prostate volume. There was improvement in maximum flow rate of 3.26 mL/s [13]. Other medications under review include cetrorelix, with some studies showing improvement in IPSS, or improvement in IPSS for larger prostates, whilst other studies showed no effect compared with placebo [14, 15]. Adverse effects included hot flushes, pain at the injection site, naso-pharyngeal inflammation and headaches [16]. Ozarelix seemed to improve the IPSS and peak urine flow rate, without impairing International Index of Erectile Function (IIEF) [17]. However, impaired libido and erectile dysfunction in short term, as well as a long term risk of reduced bone mineral density and potential ischaemic cardiac events, are important adverse effects to be borne in mind.

Hormonal agents have been directed at oestrogens as well—benzopyrans are potent, selective estrogen receptor b agonists, which induce prostatic cellular apoptosis [18]. However, no clinical outcome data is yet available.

There also exist several investigational agents, which aim to manage the secondary bladder hyperactivity component of LUTS. These include AF-353, a P2X3/P2X2/3 antagonist [19], hydroxyfasudil, a Rho-kinase inhibitor [20], WO-03028719, an oral ECE inhibitor [21] amongst others.

14.4   Laser Treatments

Several laser types and methods exist currently, aimed at reducing BPH adenoma volume. It is likely that new types of lasers, as well as new surgical techniques will be developed; with their manufacturers boasting higher efficiency with improved safety. Ideally, an affordable, simple and safe procedure will become accessible, with a simple and easy learning curve. Holmium laser enucleation of the prostate (HoLEP) was first described over 20 years ago [22], demonstrating good outflow reduction with less electrolyte disturbance compared with traditional TURP [23]. However, disadvantages include a prolonged learning curve [24] for optimal continence results and there remain risks of bleeding, sepsis and morcellation related complications such as bladder injury. Thulium lasers have also been used effectively as an enucleation technique [25].

Photosensitive vaporization of the prostate (PVP), fails to deliver tissue for histological examination. However, better perioperative outcomes can be obtained when compared with traditional monopolar TURP [26]. Will it be possible for a vaporisation technique to somehow indicate benign versus malignant prostatic pathology? It is perhaps more likely than an enucleation technique will become somewhat more automated –decreasing the surgeon's learning curve. Furthermore, a laser may have inherent properties which autodefine the correct plane for resection. It is probable that morcellation, or extraction devices will improve in their safety and efficiency levels as well (Fig. 14.1).

14.5   Ablative Treatments

Aquablation utilising the AquaBeam® (Procept Biorobotics, CA, USA) is a promising experimental modality which combines a high pressure water jet to dissect BPH tissues, with trans-rectal ultrasound guidance and a robotic hand piece (Fig. 14.2). This is a heat-free system with real time imaging using a high velocity saline jet.

Fig. 14.1 Greenlight
Laser (Courtesy of Boston
Scientific, MA, USA)

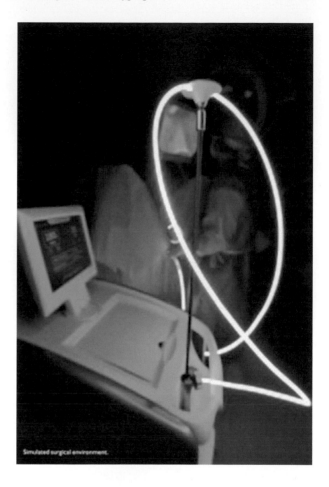

Initial safety studies have shown equivalent symptom and urodynamic outcomes
with acceptable adverse effects [27] on moderate prostate sizes up to 85 cc including many with significant middle lobes. A surgical map is manually placed to define
the resection area. The ablation time itself is low (5–12 min) in this early series,
with overall operative times (40–56 min). It is imaginable that over the next few
decades, such integration of robotics with intra-operative imaging will achieve the
aims of safer, more efficient techniques for treating BPH.

The Rezum system (NxThera, Maple Grove, MN, USA) utilizes steam convective energy to ablate BPH. Again short procedural times are of benefit (2–23 min),
with improvements in mean IPSS (23–10) and reduction in prostate volume 26% at
3 months, based on MRI [28]. A subsequent randomized trial confirms improvement of symptoms scores with mild to moderate adverse outcomes [29]. This has
been performed in an office-based setting [30] and it is predicted that more of such
technologies will be developed, able to be performed without general anaesthetic or
hospital in-patient stay.

Fig. 14.2 Aquabeam
System (Courtesy of
Procept Biorobotics, CA,
USA)

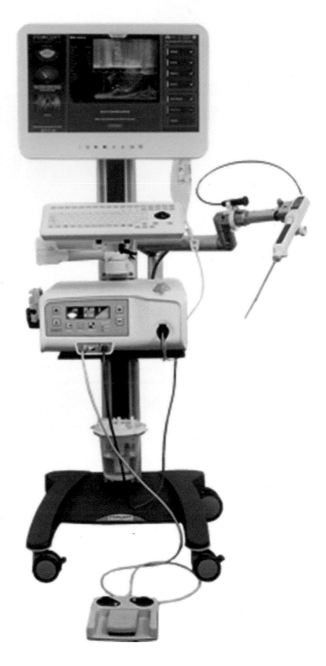

Histotripsy utilises high intensity focused ultrasound to create non thermal cavitations, resulting in a liquefied emulsion of acellular material [31]. Because the destroyed BPH is liquefied, it can drain via the urethra, as described in canine studies [32]—human trials were abandoned due to poor recruitment.

This differs from High-Intensity-Focussed Ultrasound (HiFU) in that the acoustic sound waves are converted to thermal energy, causing coagulative necrosis [33]. Several platforms are available currently, including Ablatherm® (EDAP TMS, Vaulx-en Velin, France) and the Sonoblate® (Sonacare Medical, LLC, Charlotte, NC, USA). There is some evidence to suggest improvement in symptoms scores, flow rates, albeit with possible adverse events including urinary retention, haematuria, perineal pain, sepsis [34]. However, long term follow up suggests that failure rate at 4 years is high at 44% [35].

14.6   Stents

A variety of urethral prostatic stents have been developed, trialled and abandoned over time. Although excellent in concept, they have been plagued by practical inconveniences including stent migration, storage/irritative symptoms, encrustation and need for early removal. The self expanding Urolume Wallstent® (American Medical Systems, Minnetonka, MN, USA) showed early promise however long term evaluations show only 18% of 62 patients had their stents in-situ after 12 years [36]. Furthermore, if removal was required later, resection of the overgrown urethral mucosa needs to occur, under general anaesthetic. Temporary stents avoid this—the Memotherm® metallic stent (Bard, Covington, KT, USA) has a 'memory' such that when warm water is flushed around it, the nickel–titanium alloy spiral stent becomes floppy and is easily retrieved.

To overcome some of these issues biodegradable materials are now being employed as a short-term treatment option. One example is braided polylactic-co-glycolic acid, which has been used in combination with medical treatment for men with acute urinary retention. At 1 month, 5 of 10 patients were able to void with post void residual volumes <150 mL [37]. Combinations of such treatments in the future is likely, particularly with improvements in various materials and designs of urethral stents.

14.7   Prostatic Urethral Lift

The UroLift® device (Neo Tract Inc., Pleasanton, CA, USA) relies on endoscopic placement of non-absorbable sutures attached to nitinol anchors, which retract the urethra laterally towards the prostatic capsule. Improvement in sexual health outcomes, specifically continued anterograde ejaculation, is an attractive benefit compared with other treatments for BPH, likely as the bladder neck and ejaculatory ducts are not inferred with. The procedure can be performed under local anesthetic and repeated if necessary. A meta-analysis concluded that functional and symptom outcomes were improved at 12 months, however prostate volume <80 cc was an inclusion criteria and a lack of a middle lobe recommended. An additional benefit of the Urolift is the relative preservation of ejaculatory function, presumably due to

Fig. 14.3 The Urolift
Device (Courtesy of
NeoTract Inc., CA, USA)

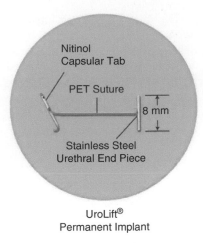

the preservation of native prostatic tissue. The more common early (within 3 months) complications included dysuria (25–53%), haematuria (16–75%), pelvic pain (3.7–19.3%), urgency (7.8–10%), transient incontinence (1.9–16%) as well as urinary tract infection (3.2–10%) [38]. Long-term data is pending but it is possible with proven results that the current maximum prostate size will be increased to above 100 cc widening patient access and improving uptake. The ability to perform a secondary procedure on men who have undergone Urolift is also a potential difficulty which requires evaluation (Fig. 14.3).

14.8 Nanorobotics

The future surgical tool will likely become much smaller, nano to be precise. Nanorobotics refers to microscopic machines or robots. These devices would enable non-invasive treatments to be directed at specific organs, or even at specific cells. A cloud-like theory has been suggested [39] whereby, due to the tiny nature of each individual nanorobot, many would be required to act in tandem to perform a specific function. No clinical application yet exists, but it is certainly a concept for the future that could act at a cellular level to reduce BPH. Being non-invasive, surgical complications would be reduced or even eliminated. The cost of such technology, like all innovations, would in time likely become cheaper as well.

14.9 Conclusion

Many treatments exist to treat significant BPH, however, they are all imperfect. We have and will continue to develop and improve our options—the holy grail being an effective, safe and economical treatment. It is highly possible, that resectoscopes, lasers, stents and even medications may ultimately be placed upon the shelf of surgical museums, once a non-invasive, complication free, effective treatment arises. Whether this will be the nano-robot, or the magic-bullet pharma-innovation, or perhaps, something else entirely only the future will tell.

References

1. World Report on Ageing and Health. Geneva: WHO; 2015.
2. Filson CP, Wei JT, Hollingsworth JM. Trends in medical management of men with lower urinary tract symptoms suggestive of benign prostatic hyperplasia. Urology. 2013;82(6):1386–92.
3. Cindolo L, Pirozzi L, Fanizza C, Romero M, Sountoulides P, Roehrborn CG, et al. Actual medical management of lower urinary tract symptoms related to benign prostatic hyperplasia: temporal trends of prescription and hospitalization rates over 5 years in a large population of Italian men. Int Urol Nephrol. 2014;46(4):695–701.
4. Ingimarsson JP, Isaksson HJ, Sigbjarnarson HP, Gudmundsson J, Geirsson G. Increased population use of medications for male lower urinary tract symptoms/benign prostatic hyperplasia correlates with changes in indications for transurethral resection of the prostate. Scand J Urol. 2014;48(1):73–8.
5. Djavan B, Chapple C, Milani S, Marberger M. State of the art on the efficacy and tolerability of alpha1-adrenoceptor antagonists in patients with lower urinary tract symptoms suggestive of benign prostatic hyperplasia. Urology. 2004;64(6):1081–8.
6. Kojima Y, Sasaki S, Hayashi Y, Tsujimoto G, Kohri K. Subtypes of α1-adrenoceptors in BPH: future prospects for personalized medicine. Nat Clin Pract Urol. 2009;6(1):44–53.
7. McConnell JD, Roehrborn CG, Bautista OM, Andriole GL Jr, Dixon CM, Kusek JW, et al. The long-term effect of doxazosin, finasteride, and combination therapy on the clinical progression of benign prostatic hyperplasia. N Engl J Med. 2003;349(25):2387–98.
8. Roehrborn CG, Siami P, Barkin J, Damiao R, Major-Walker K, Nandy I, et al. The effects of combination therapy with dutasteride and tamsulosin on clinical outcomes in men with symptomatic benign prostatic hyperplasia: 4-year results from the CombAT study. Eur Urol. 2010;57(1):123–31.
9. Shore N. NX-1207: a novel investigational drug for the treatment of benign prostatic hyperplasia. Expert Opin Investig Drugs. 2010;19(2):305–10.
10. Williams SA, Merchant RF, Garrett-Mayer E, Isaacs JT, Buckley JT, Denmeade SR. A prostate-specific antigen-activated channel-forming toxin as therapy for prostatic disease. J Natl Cancer Inst. 2007;99(5):376–85.
11. Denmeade SR, Egerdie B, Steinhoff G, Merchant R, Abi-Habib R, Pommerville P. Phase 1 and 2 studies demonstrate the safety and efficacy of intraprostatic injection of PRX302 for the targeted treatment of lower urinary tract symptoms secondary to benign prostatic hyperplasia. Eur Urol. 2011;59(5):747–54.
12. Adorini L, Penna G, Amuchastegui S, Cossetti C, Aquilano F, Mariani R, et al. Inhibition of prostate growth and inflammation by the vitamin D receptor agonist BXL-628 (elocalcitol). J Steroid Biochem Mol Biol. 2007;103(3–5):689–93.
13. Penna G, Fibbi B, Amuchastegui S, Corsiero E, Laverny G, Silvestrini E, et al. The vitamin D receptor agonist elocalcitol inhibits IL-8-dependent benign prostatic hyperplasia stromal cell proliferation and inflammatory response by targeting the RhoA/Rho kinase and NF-kappaB pathways. Prostate. 2009;69(5):480–93.
14. Colli E, Rigatti P, Montorsi F, Artibani W, Petta S, Mondaini N, et al. BXL628, a novel vitamin D3 analog arrests prostate growth in patients with benign prostatic hyperplasia: a randomized clinical trial. Eur Urol. 2006;49(1):82–6.
15. Maclean C LF, Drewe J, Dzmitryieu AV, Gres A, Strockyi A, Dovger V, Ulys A, Cerniauskienè A, Geavlete P, Nikolovski M. Efficacy and safety of Teverelix LA, A new GNRH antagonist in patients with benign prostatic hyperplasia (BPH). Results from a phase II randomized, double-blind, placebo-controlled, multicentre, multinational study investigating two sin-

gle injections of 60mg at 48 hours interval administered s.c. to treatment naive patients suffering from BPH. Eur Urol Suppl. 2007;6(2):109.

16. Debruyne F, Gres AA, Arustamov DL. Placebo-controlled dose-ranging phase 2 study of subcutaneously administered LHRH antagonist cetrorelix in patients with symptomatic benign prostatic hyperplasia. Eur Urol. 2008;54(1):170–7.

17. Debruyne FMJ. The efficacy and safety of ozarelix, a novel GnRH antagonist, in men with lower urinary tract symptoms (LUTS) due to benign prostatic hyperplasia (BPH). J Urol. 2007;177(Suppl):512.

18. Norman BH, Dodge JA, Richardson TI, Borromeo PS, Lugar CW, Jones SA, et al. Benzopyrans are selective estrogen receptor beta agonists with novel activity in models of benign prostatic hyperplasia. J Med Chem. 2006;49(21):6155–7.

19. Munoz A, Somogyi GT, Boone TB, Ford AP, Smith CP. Modulation of bladder afferent signals in normal and spinal cord-injured rats by purinergic P2X3 and P2X2/3 receptors. BJU Int. 2012;110(8 Pt B):E409–14.

20. Inoue S, Saito M, Takenaka A. Hydroxyfasudil ameliorates bladder dysfunction in male spontaneously hypertensive rats. Urology. 2012;79(5):1186e9–14.

21. Schroder A, Tajimi M, Matsumoto H, Schroder C, Brands M, Andersson KE. Protective effect of an oral endothelin converting enzyme inhibitor on rat detrusor function after outlet obstruction. J Urol. 2004;172(3):1171–4.

22. Gilling PJ, Cass CB, Malcolm AR, Fraundorfer MR. Combination holmium and Nd:YAG laser ablation of the prostate: initial clinical experience. J Endourol. 1995;9(2):151–3.

23. Chilton CP, Mundy IP, Wiseman O. Results of holmium laser resection of the prostate for benign prostatic hyperplasia. J Endourol. 2000;14(6):533–4.

24. Robert G, Cornu JN, Fourmarier M, Saussine C, Descazeaud A, Azzouzi AR, et al. Multicentre prospective evaluation of the learning curve of holmium laser enucleation of the prostate (HoLEP). BJU Int. 2016;117(3):495–9.

25. Kuo RL, Kim SC, Lingeman JE, Paterson RF, Watkins SL, Simmons GR, et al. Holmium laser enucleation of prostate (HoLEP): the Methodist Hospital experience with greater than 75 gram enucleations. J Urol. 2003;170(1):149–52.

26. Cornu JN, Ahyai S, Bachmann A, de la Rosette J, Gilling P, Gratzke C, et al. A systematic review and meta-analysis of functional outcomes and complications following transurethral procedures for lower urinary tract symptoms resulting from benign prostatic obstruction: an update. Eur Urol. 2015;67(6):1066–96.

27. Gilling P, Reuther R, Kahokehr A, Fraundorfer M. Aquablation—image-guided robot-assisted waterjet ablation of the prostate: initial clinical experience. BJU Int. 2016;117(6):923–9.

28. Dixon CCE, Pacik D. PD26-09 transurethral water vapor therapy for BPH; 1-year clinical results of the first-in-man and Rezum I clinical trials using the Rezum system. J Urol. 2014;191(4):e762.

29. McVary KT, Gange SN, Gittelman MC, Goldberg KA, Patel K, Shore ND, et al. Minimally invasive prostate convective water vapor energy ablation: a multicenter, randomized, controlled study for the treatment of lower urinary tract symptoms secondary to benign prostatic hyperplasia. J Urol. 2016;195(5):1529–38.

30. Wagrell LTM. Transurethral convective water vapor ablation therapy for BPH; a single center's experience using the Rezum system in an office-based setting. J Urol. 2014;191(4s):e762.

31. Roberts WW, Hall TL, Ives K, Wolf JS Jr, Fowlkes JB, Cain CA. Pulsed cavitational ultrasound: a noninvasive technology for controlled tissue ablation (histotripsy) in the rabbit kidney. J Urol. 2006;175(2):734–8.

32. Lake AM, Hall TL, Kieran K, Fowlkes JB, Cain CA, Roberts WW. Histotripsy: minimally invasive technology for prostatic tissue ablation in an in vivo canine model. Urology. 2008;72(3):682–6.

33. Madersbacher S, Kratzik C, Susani M, Marberger M. Tissue ablation in benign prostatic hyperplasia with high intensity focused ultrasound. J Urol. 1994;152(6 Pt 1):1956–60. discussion 60-1

34. Sullivan L, Casey RW, Pommerville PJ, Marich KW. Canadian experience with high intensity focused ultrasound for the treatment of BPH. Can J Urol. 1999;6(3):799–805.
35. Madersbacher S, Schatzl G, Djavan B, Stulnig T, Marberger M. Long-term outcome of transrectal high- intensity focused ultrasound therapy for benign prostatic hyperplasia. Eur Urol. 2000;37(6):687–94.
36. Masood S, Djaladat H, Kouriefs C, Keen M, Palmer JH. The 12-year outcome analysis of an endourethral wallstent for treating benign prostatic hyperplasia. BJU Int. 2004;94(9):1271–4.
37. Kotsar A, Isotalo T, Juuti H, Mikkonen J, Leppiniemi J, Hanninen V, et al. Biodegradable braided poly(lactic-co-glycolic acid) urethral stent combined with dutasteride in the treatment of acute urinary retention due to benign prostatic enlargement: a pilot study. BJU Int. 2009;103(5):626–9.
38. Perera M, Roberts MJ, Doi SA, Bolton D. Prostatic urethral lift improves urinary symptoms and flow while preserving sexual function for men with benign prostatic hyperplasia: a systematic review and meta-analysis. Eur Urol. 2015;67(4):704–13.
39. Mali S. Nanorobots: changing face of healthcare system. J Biomed Eng. 2014;1(3):1012.

Index

© Springer International Publishing AG 2018
V. Kasivisvanathan, B. Challacombe (eds.), *The Big Prostate*,
https://doi.org/10.1007/978-3-319-64704-3

Printed by Printforce, the Netherlands

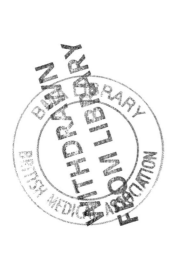